International Perspectives on Long-Term Care

International Perspectives on Long-Term Care

Laura Reif, PhD
Brahna Trager, ACSW, LCSW
Editors

The Haworth Press
New York

International Perspectives on Long-Term Care has also been published as *Home Health Care Services Quarterly,* Volume 5, Numbers 3/4, Fall 1984/Winter 1984/85.

The Haworth Press, Inc., 28 East 22 Street, New York, NY 10010

Library of Congress Cataloging in Publication Data
Main entry under title:

International perspectives on long-term care.

    "Has also been published as Home health care services quarterly, volume 5, number 3/4, fall/winter 1984"—T.p. verso.
    Includes bibliographies.
    1. Long-term care of the sick—Addresses, essays, lectures. 2. Aged—Home care—Addresses, essays, lectures. 3. Aged—Medical care—Addresses, essays, lectures. I. Reif, Laura. II. Trager, Brahna. [DNLM: 1. Cross–Cultural Comparison. 2. Long Term Care—in old age. W1 H0502R v.5 no.3/4 / WT 30 I635]
RA644.5.I58 1985   362.1'4   85-8442
ISBN 0-86656-400-4
ISBN 0-86656-445-4 (pbk.)

International Perspectives on Long-Term Care

Home Health Care Services Quarterly
Volume 5, Numbers 3/4

CONTENTS

JANET E. STARR, BS. *Executive Director, Home Care Association of New York State, Inc., Syracuse, New York*

MONNICA C. STEWART, MB, BS, D(Obst), RCOG, *Community Medicine Physician, City and East London Area Health Authority, London, United Kingdom*

ANN-MARIE THOM, *Executive Director, Visiting Nurse Association of New York, New York*

PATRICIA THOMAS, *Executive Director, Visiting Homemakers Association, Toronto, Ontario, Canada*

JUDITH LA VOR WILLIAMS, *Florence Heller School for Advanced Studies in Social Welfare, Brandeis University, Waltham, Massachusetts*

International Perspectives on Long-Term Care

INTRODUCTION

Issues in Long-Term Care: An International Perspective

Brahna Trager, ACSW, LCSW

Longer life, viewed in some cultures as a prime achievement of civilized progress, and in others as a problem which bodes ill for the economic future, is nevertheless a demographic fact, at least in the developed countries, and in projection, in the developing countries as well. In different degrees, all populations are experiencing demographic changes, affected by a combination of factors such as successive wars, natural disasters, inadequate resources in some countries, and in others by economic development, by technological advances, and an improved life style.

As there are national differences in the view of these changes, there are also differences in the view of their implications for public policy, and even of the perception of the relative importance of the place which such change should occupy in the development of public policy. What may be a matter of pride in one country (the reduction of infant mortality and the addition of years to the human life span), evidence that overall a population which is as healthy as it can be and therefore a national asset, may, in another country, be seen as projecting an economic burden. Differences in national tradition are also factors. Established family policy coupled with practical understanding of the changed structure of modern family life may be contrasted with a sentimentalized version of the family as inde-

1

pendently responsible for its members, bound to sacrifice by ties of affection and loyalty regardless of the most destructive external circumstances. The older cultures tend to view the national good and the "personal good" as inextricably bound together. History has taught that the values of an egalitarian approach to public well-being may be ignored in the short run; enlightened self-interest has taught that in the long run the benefits of humanism far outweigh the potential disadvantages of public indifference.

Whatever the causes, most of the Western European countries, and developed countries which have followed their systems, have supported broad social policy and have, to a significant extent, implemented such policy on behalf of the aging with extensive, accessible and generally effective health and social programs. The changes in the composition of their populations which have stimulated the extension of services and entitlements to their longer lived members have not evoked popular pressure to restrict or reduce these services and entitlements. Rather they have stimulated efforts to meet new need practically and, perhaps with increased humanism. The international literature makes increasing reference to the "quality of life," to, as Terroir[1] so aptly phrases it "assuring that population the medical and social care which it requires to preserve an independent place in society . . . (and) during the last years of life . . . a right to a life in society which provides as much warmth as possible."

If there is very little indication that systems of health and social care in these countries are in danger of being dismantled, there is marked evidence that long-term care systems and services are being studied attentively with a view to making them more effective, more responsive, more acceptable, and perhaps even less costly in economic terms. Most of these countries have had long-standing programs for the protection of the health of their childhood populations, and medical protection has been available either as insurance or in national systems of health protection against normal risks—protection against acute health problems. The development of long-term care, however, has presented problems which have challenged existing patterns of care for older people—often excellent institutional facilities conforming to misguided ideas about the ideal living situation and service requirements of old and very old people. Demographic studies which project[2] growth in the older population—particularly in that sector which in France is often referred to as the "fourth age" have stimulated increased emphasis on planning of care more realistically adapted to the needs of these populations. This attention has been influenced by biological research on aging and by rather extensive inquiry into the desires of older consumers themselves, through polls, through household interviews and through review of existing systems with regard to their effectiveness and their acceptability. Assumptions about aging are changing with research: the assumption that physical and cognitive function must inevitably deteriorate with advancing age appears to be less reliable, with indications that most people who reach and pass retirement age do not change radically,[3] that given the right circumstances intellectual growth may continue and that physical impairment when it occurs is related to disease. The phrase "aging is not a disease" is becoming more current. Extreme old age does, however, present a challenge to guarantees of a "right to life in society." For these groups and for older people with varying degrees of functional and physiological limitation, the need for changes in policy and systems of service delivery is being recognized. This need for change has been further strengthened by an increasingly vocal population—the aging themselves. For the most part they appear, in all cultures, to reject the idea of segregation, of institutions, however well equipped they may be, in favor of continuity in their life style, preferably in their habitual environment. What has been occurring in these countries, therefore, is a major shift away from institutional solutions to a more attentive and practical tailoring of programs and services to people with diminished capacity. This has been accompanied by augmentation of economic support, adaptation of existing housing and/or construction of housing which allows for maximum independence. A very broad range of support services is being developed and made available. Innovative methods of service delivery are being tested in studies which are, perhaps, less "research oriented" and more practical than the "project" approach which has been so prevalent in the United States in recent years.[4] Although institutions remain a part of the service range in all countries, more selective admission is being envisioned and those which remain are being "humanized" in order to reduce the sterility of life in them, and where health services are deficient, these are being added with efforts to strengthen the linkage with mainstream medical care. The major emphasis appears to be in the direction of community care, and since this requires a range of services which will make life in the community feasible at least and desirable at best, existing resources are being extended and new combinations of services are being developed. There appears to be evidence that the strongest movement in long-term care will be in the direction of what, in Sweden, has been called "normalization" of the care of the elderly, that is, continued life in the personal environment wherever that is possible, and where it is not, in an environment as close to normal life as possible.

THE FAMILY

There is a range in public policy approaches to the role of the family in the provision of long-term care. The least realistic public policy consists of strong sentiment and minimal action. The most practical public policy consists of factual analysis and the development of public programs which support (or replace, if necessary) family efforts in long-term care. Beginning in the 1960's, research indicated that the family role in long-term care remains important and the family contribution substantial.[5] In the least developed public policy vis-à-vis the role of the family, reluctance to support family effort ranges from expressed fear that assistance will tend to "dry up" the will of the family to fulfill what is considered its moral obligation, to a kind of laissez-faire based on the assumption that the family exists (ignoring statistics concerning the absence of family in the elderly), and will perform that role well or badly. There is ample evidence in the literature concerning the family in long-term care, of the tragedy that this latter assumption imposes on the individuals involved and on the fabric of family relationships. There is also evidence that delayed intervention may create problems which might be avoided and in the long run results in more costly care measures.

In the more practical, and more enlightened approach to the family in long-term care, public responsibility is assumed, based on recognition of such factors as shifts in economic pressures affecting the family structure, with the result that family members are entering the work force in increasing numbers, the effect on the composition of the family with increased longevity in its oldest members and pressure on potential caregivers who are also entering the older age ranges and the fact, as has been pointed out in recent studies[6] that the population of the consumer group which is most in need of long-term care is composed almost entirely of women who are alone, either widowed, without living family members, never married and without the so-called "informal" care network which is frequently cited as a resource.

Enlightened public policy in countries with more developed care systems is therefore directed to providing at public expense, assistance to the family when necessary in order to preserve, for as long as possible, its potential for partial or full support thus avoiding the need for measures which destroy supportive and practical relationships in long-term care. These measures take the form of payment to family members who are then able to remain at home to provide long-term care substituting this income for income from outside employment; it has provided in legislation and public budgets, adapted housing which provides for more convenient home care, or for maximum proximity of family members so that there will be greater ease in communication, support and the provision of assistance; it has recognized the pressures of such care on the physical and emotional reserves of family members and has developed a range of home delivered services, the most wanted of which has been household assistance and personal care from paraprofessionals who, in most countries, have been trained to provide practical assistance but who are also able to offer more specialized services usually assumed by professionals in the United States. The range of organized community services which have been made available in order to implement care in the community are by now well known and are beginning to be seen as resources which it might be profitable to develop in the United States. These, however, are provided in most countries to families—an important distinction since it does not assume that the family, if there is one, will assume full responsibility for long-term care. For those who are alone, family policy, it appears, continues to operate. Most countries are beginning to turn away from the institution as the inevitable solution. The same approaches are being undertaken, namely recognition that the familiar environment should be maintained, or something as close to that environment as possible. The most impressive part of this latter approach is the recognition that all individuals have had a family history and that attachment to the familiar is an important and therapeutic part of life when the representatives of family warmth and family support may no longer be present; a recognition of the value of continuity in the human life experience, which in the case of the elderly becomes as important as the need for security in early childhood. A recent comparative study of the elderly in London and the elderly in New York[7] bears out this fact: older people in London feel more "secure" in the knowledge that there is assured public support if and when it becomes necessary than does a similar group in New York. This is an intangible yet probably a most valuable evidence of the "humanisation" of public policy in these countries.

ORGANIZATION AND ADMINISTRATION

Most long-term care in the developed countries has had the advantage of pre-existing programs for the general population to which entitlement has been established for many years (relatively generous social security provision, health care, economic supplements for special groups and for special needs).

The care requirements of the growing population in the older age ranges in these countries, therefore, have had the advantage of an established base in public service coupled with a relatively responsive public attitude with respect to the extension of services to the older population. Since acute care is generally available it appeared initially that some extension of existing services to older people would provide long-term care: more in-patient facilities, more old peoples' homes, innovation in the form of retirement villages similar to those provided for the handicapped,[8] and provisions similar to those provided for disabled veterans; transportation privileges, provision for attendant care. Shifts in understanding coupled,

with increased pressure on these resources, have brought
about major changes in public policy, and with these changes,
weaknesses in the established mechanisms for the organization, administration and funding of service systems have become apparent. Obstacles to service distribution, to coordination, to smoothly orchestrated linkages between the various
public and private authorities appear to be inherent in the
way they have traditionally developed and this has been most
apparent in long-term care, and more particularly in long-
term care in the community which is intended to implement
the shift away from the institution to the personal environment. In more advanced systems, such as Sweden and the UK
for example, the availability of resources does not automati-
cally guarantee comprehensive services even when they are
publicly funded. As in the United States, difficulties arise
when the needed components of care are organized, administered and funded by different levels of government (local authority, county, region, central government) and by a variety
of private-public arrangements. In some instances the needs
of the older population are understood to be different in kind
and in quality from those of the general population and the
response has been the creation of special government authorities directed exclusively to the needs of the aging population,
and in some instances what appear to be separate delivery
systems are being developed, which, while they do emphasize
the special needs of the group for which they are intended,
may also have the potential of segregating the elderly population in policy and service consideration, an effect which may
ultimately work to the disadvantage of this population. In the
UK, for example, this approach has been discussed with respect to the pros and cons of special Geriatric in-patient units:

—A second pattern is for the geriatric unit to provide an
   age defined service taking all patients above a certain
   age, usually either 65 of 75.
—A third pattern is to integrate medical facilities for the
   elderly with those for all other age groups with admission
   units run by teams of consultants, each team containing a
   specialist in geriatric medicine.
——In choosing between these patterns several considerations are involved. Most important is the quality of care

provided for the patient and the . . . pattern in which the . . . care of an elderly patient is managed by doctors who have no responsibility for providing longer term care . . . is clearly unsatisfactory. Nothing improves a doctor's knowledge and skill and administrative expertise as much as the responsibility for looking after his own mistakes and seeing the longer-term effects of his care . . .

— A third problem raised by the age-defined specialty is that it does not make biological sense. Human adult aging is a continuous exponential process and most of the diseases of old age have their origins earlier in life . . .

— Doctors interested in researching into the diseases of old age need access to patients of younger ages if advances are to be made in understanding the natural history of disease and its prevention.[9]

These considerations have more general application. Similar problems are presented by the separation of responsibility for in-patient care and community care. Hospital social workers, for example, when they are responsible for discharge planning have described the difficulties encountered when they are unable to have close contact with community services and better understanding of the environment to which the patient will go.

Almost without exception countries make a distinction between what is considered "health" care and what is considered "social" care. Unlike the United States where "social" usually carries the connotation of means-tested services to a poverty level group, the distinction in other countries is still complex and cumbersome. Medical care is clearly defined, and since entitlement is established, funding may not be a problem. The distinction between what is directly provided in a hospital or by a physician in the community and that range of services included under the conception of "social care," the latter providing services which might logically be considered health services is compounded by the fact that they are provided at different government levels and from different funding sources, usually with different requirements. While substantial public funding may be invested in social care, it may, in some instances, be means-tested in some countries. This, however, is not the major problem. The major problem is in achieving comprehensiveness and coordination when there is a need for multiple services:

> The services which are required to meet . . . needs are organizationally highly fragmented coming from a wide range of sources, both formal and informal. The picture of resource provision . . . is all to often that of a series of piecemeal interventions by a range of actors, none of whom have a clear responsibility for taking a broader overview of need.

> " . . . Each level has full control of the policy which it expects to implement. . . . Because spheres of control are precisely defined there are . . . no situations in which common agreements are made. . . . Dependent old people find themselves on the borders of these respective spheres because their need is for care which is "medico-social."[10]

Organized voluntary programs are important in all countries although their roles may differ. They function primarily in the "social" sphere, although many of them provide health care personnel and offer health services. In some countries, as in France, the role of the "associations" may be far more than a contributing supplementary one. Powerful federations of associations may function as advocates, exert considerable influence on legislation, organize and provide a wide range of services and programs and occupy a quasi-public position as recipients and distributors of public money for publicly funded services.[11] The same separation between "medical" and "social" care may also exist complicated by fragmentation within the organizations.

In the developed countries it is apparent that, while resources for "social" care are not unlimited, they are available in far greater supply proportionately than they are in the United States. What is more important, however, is that there is a very broad view of what people in need of long-term care in the community require, and the assumption that provision of an extensive range of services is appropriately a public responsibility. Administrative and organizational difficulties around the bridging of "health-social" distinctions may be easier to resolve when linkage to economic and social class are not the prime consideration. Implementation of administrative mechanisms which recognize the multi-faceted needs of people in need of long-term care in the community appears to have a relatively high priority in these countries.

COSTS

The costs of long-term care have not, until relatively recently, been a central issue in most developed countries. (In the developing countries, the inability to fund adequate health care for total populations remains a continuing problem; long life, and consequently the need for long-term care, are not a part of considerations in health care provision—the control of infant mortality and the provision of a minimally improved life style are central and crucial to these countries.)

Although the percentage of the GNP for health care expenditures in most developed countries has been approximately the same (around 9% with the exception of the UK—5.8% and Canada—7.4%, which have kept relatively stable in the years 1975–1980),[12] the inclusive percentage figure is less significant in consideration of the costs of long-term care than the fact that the proportion of expenditures for health care for older sections of the population have increased, and, as in the United States, health care expenditures are attributed to a relatively small segment of the older population. Concerns in other ways are similar to those in the United States. There has been bed blocking in acute care institutions with very little new hospital construction, and acute care beds are occupied by people whose real need is for a different level of care. Length of stay in acute care beds differs in different countries, but extended stays are not unusual. Nevertheless, although concern with costs is appearing more frequently in the literature, there does not appear to be the same driving concern with costs and cost control as is apparent in the United States, in spite of the fact that some of the Western European countries have larger percentages of older people in their populations than does the United States. There is, in most countries a trend toward the re-structuring of health care delivery systems, with efforts to arrive at care which, while it may also result in cost reduction, will be more compatible with the what consumers appear to want—care in the community which provides security and is effective. There is increasing emphasis on community health centers which offer multiple services and emphasize team interaction; the UK has also begun a restructuring of its health care management system in an effort to tighten control and increase efficiency;[13] it may be effective, it may also simply insert another level of non-service personnel; in general, however, most countries appear to be placing greater emphasis on home care and housing arrangements which will delay or avoid hospitalization, or failing that, reduction of hospitalization by providing part-time in-patient care. France, the UK and Canada have been developing "hospital-at-home" programs and in several countries coordination is being encouraged through the use of multiservice assessment teams, and community or regional coordinators. Most countries appear to recognize the need for increased service personnel at the community level.[14]

It might be said that a review of international approaches to the provision of long-term care will be of little assistance unless it can be accompanied by such things as cost comparisons, hard data about utilization, and the evidence which supports conclusions about effectiveness in other systems. It might also be said that inordinate amounts of research invested in determining cost-effectiveness could also be self-defeating. The involved population is not simply a theater for research; it is important to view the need as a human need, and there is value in reviews which provide innovative and imaginative information about solutions to human problems in other countries. In the area of community care which is relatively new and limited in its scope in the United States such solutions offer considerable opportunity for thought and, it is hoped, some degree of emulation.

REFERENCES

1. Terroir, Patrick. "Report of a Mission to Review Care Provided to the Aged in Sweden." Home Health Care Services Quarterly, 5 (Fall/Winter, 1984).
2. The Aging World (Chapter Two) in *Aging in all nations. A special report on the United Nations World Assembly on Aging.* Vienna, Austria July 26-August 6, 1982. The National Council on Aging Inc. Prepared by William E. Oriol.

3. Butler, Lewis H. and Newacheck, Paul W. Health and Social Factors Relevant to Long-term Care Policy. Chapter two. In *Policy Options in Long-term Care.* Edited by Judith Meltzer, Frank Farrow and Harold Richman. The University of Chicago Press, 1981.

4. Trager, Brahna. In *Place of Policy: Public Adventures in Non-Institutional Long-term Care.* Presented at the American Public Health Association National Conference, 1981. Unpublished.

5. Shanas, Ethel, et al. *Old People in Three Industrial Societies.* New York. Atherton, 1968; and Roussel, Louis. *La Famille Après le Mariage des Enfants. Etude des Relations entre Générations.* Cahier no. 78. Presses Universitaires de France, 1976.

6. Collot, Claudette; Florea, Aurelia; Jani-le Bris; Naegele, Gerhard; Plum, Wolfgang; Ridoux, Ann; Turrini, Olga. *The Social Situation of Older Women Living Alone in Three European Countries.* Collection "CLEIRPPA," 1982. Paris, France; and Brody, Elaine M. "Women in the Middle and Family Help to Older People." *The Gerontologist,* 21 (October 1981) 471–480.

7. Gurland, Barry; Copeland, John; and Colleagues. *The Mind and Mood of Aging: Mental Health Problems of the Community Elderly in New York and London.* The Haworth Press, New York, 1983.

8. De Jong, Gerben. *Independent Living and Disability Policy in the Netherlands: Three Models of Residential Care and Independent Living.* World Rehabilitation Fund. New York, 1983.

9. Grimsley-Evans, J., Great Britain, pp. 47–48 in *Hospitalization of the Elderly: An International Perspective.* International Center of Social Gerontology. Paris, France, 1980.

10. Terroir, Patrick. Op. cit.

11. Schorr, Alvin L. Social Security and Social Services in France. U.S. Department of Health, Education and Welfare. Social Security Administration. Division of Research and Statistics. Research Report No. 7, 1965.

12. Nusberg, Charlotte. The Impact of Aging Populations on Health Care Budgets: Part II. *Aging International,* Winter 1983/4.

13. Department of Health and Social Security. London. *Health Services Management.* Implementation of the NHS Management Inquiry Report, 1984.

14. Hospitals-at-Home in France and Canada. *Ageing International,* Spring, 1984; Santé des Personnes Agées. Assises Nationales des Retraités et Personnes Agées. Secretariat d'Etat Chargé des Personnes Agées Ministère des Affaires Sociales et de la Solidarité Nationale, Paris, France, 1983.

Home Health Services
for the Elderly:
The English Way

Daniel I. Zwick, MA

ABSTRACT. Strengthening home health and related community services for the care of the elderly at home has received
high priority in policy statements on the National Health Service. Findings from a series of recent studies and reports on
these issues are reviewed, highlighting accomplishments and
problems of primary health care teams, especially the district
nurses, and the many other contributing community services.
Seven lessons are discussed, emphasizing the relationships
among home health and other community services, the importance of voluntary services, the impact of hospital and psychiatric services, needs for special training, difficulties of cost
analyses, and the slow pace of progress.

England has an extensive system and a long history of
home health services. These activities have been emphasized
for over a century (Abel-Smith, 1960; Merry, 1960). Public
policies have repeatedly given priority to the provision of services in the community and home to the elderly and others.

A review of these experiences is timely. In the last few
years, a series of studies of community care has been made by
public and private groups in England. These analyses document past accomplishments and problems, current activities
and future prospects.

While health programs are seldom transferable in a simple
way from one country to another, in considering the English
experiences, we can gain some perspective on the potentiali-

Daniel I. Zwick is a consultant on health policy. He was with the U.S. Department of Health and Human Services and the Office of Economic Opportunity in a
number of health management, planning and evaluation positions. His current address is 6508 Bannockburn Drive, Bethesda, Maryland 20817.

ties and difficulties of undertaking further activities along these lines. We may also learn the extent to which expectations and goals set forth for these services are likely to be achievable and realistic. Such lessons can help us advance the American way.

This paper has two major parts. The first describes the organization and scope of home health care and related services for the elderly in England. Particular attention is given to the primary health care team and nursing services. Readers who are very familiar with the English health care system may wish to skip or skim this section and focus on the second part.

Part two discusses seven major lessons which I have identified in reviewing these experiences. While other reviewers might highlight other aspects of this complex field, I believe these seven points are critical to any consideration of these issues. The paper is based on a visit to England in the spring of 1982 and review of the pertinent publications.

Our interest in the English approach was intensified by a number of reported observations about its operations. An English writer (Brockelhurst, 1975, p. 39) points out: "every attempt is made to support people in their own homes and this is successful to a remarkable extent." Two American researchers (Kane & Kane, 1980, p. 26) note; "one can not help but be impressed that in Britain large numbers of quite infirm persons were being maintained in their own homes." On the other hand, we are warned (Pinker, 1980, p. 283) that: "long-term care needs of the elderly infirm (could) lead to a breakdown of our present health services."

SOME BACKGROUND DATA

Comparisons of health care data on an international basis are difficult and dangerous. Definitions and collection systems vary greatly. However, some comparisons may be suggestive even though they are presented—and should be used—with caution.

The elderly population is growing relatively rapidly in England, as in the U.S. About 15 percent of the English population is 65 years of age or older, compared to about 11 percent in the U.S.. . . . The largest percentage increase is among persons 75 years and older; the very elderly (85 years and older) are likely to increase by a third during the 1980s.

About 95 percent of those 65 years and over live at home in England. About 30 percent live alone. The ratio of the very old who are incapacitated and living alone has been increasing.

Life expectancy at birth is similar in England and the U.S. In 1978, it was 70.2 years in England and 69.5 years in the U.S. for males. For females, the respective figures were 76.3 and 77.2 years.

Health care expenditures in England approximate 6 percent of the national wealth; the comparable U.S. figure is about 10 percent. Spending for the National Health Service (NHS) accounts for about 11 percent of public outlays; a similar portion of the U.S. national budget is devoted to health services. Expenditures in England for those age 75 and over is almost six times greater than those 16–64 years of age. Expenditures for community health services, exclusive of physician services, has been between six and seven percent of NHS outlays. In England also health budgets have been severely constrained in recent years due to limited growth and strains in the general economy.

In 1978, there were about 13 physicians and 30 registered nurses for every 10,000 persons in England. In the U.S., there are about 19 physicians and 40 registered nurses per 10,000. There are about five general practitioners (GPs) for every 10,000 persons in England compared to about three physicians in general or family practice (and seven in primary care practice) per 10,000 in the U.S.

Hospital admissions appear to be at a much lower rate in England. The Department of Health and Social Security (DHSS) reported in 1980 that about 100 of every 1000 persons are admitted to a hospital annually for acute care; for persons 65 and older, the rate is about 170 per 1000. Reported hospitalization rates in U.S. short-stay hospitals are about 160 per 1000 for all ages and 390 per 1000 for those 65 years and over (Department of Health and Human Services, 1981).

On the other hand, stays in English hospitals seem to be longer than in the U.S. . . . They average between nine and ten days for acute conditions, compared to less than eight days in the U.S. In both countries, stays have been decreasing markedly.

Health districts are the local units for managing health services in the NHS. There are about 190 districts, with an average population of about 250,000 persons. There are, of course, no comparable units in the U.S.; the closest comparison may be the approximately 200 local health planning areas which have an average population of over a million persons.

It has been estimated (Kane & Kane, 1980, p.5) that an average health district includes:

—35,000 persons over the age of 65,
—4,500 elderly appreciably or severely handicapped,
—800 elderly in old-age homes,
—800 elderly receiving hospital care, and
—1000 elderly requiring domiciliary care.

Services for the elderly use a large share of both outpatient and inpatient resources in almost all health districts.

POLICIES AND PRIORITIES

In 1976 the first effort was made to establish rational and systematic priorities for the NHS. "Priorities for Health and Personal Social Services in England" was issued by the DHSS for consideration and comment. The statement highlights the pressures on health resources and the necessity for hard choices (p. 8):

> As knowledge advances and skills improve, the services are able to do more and the public expects more to be done. Standards of need tend to be relative and what is reasonable at any given time depends on what the country can afford and is willing to pay for as well as on professional assessments of need. As a result there is likely to be a gap between the services which are provided and the demands made upon them. Difficult choices have to be made to decide how far particular demands should be met. These choices are particularly hard when there can only be a slow rate of growth in resources.

Within this context, high priority for the expansion of primary care services in the community is proposed. An increase of 3.8 percent a year is set for primary care services, although a total growth rate of only 2 percent a year is projected. Community nursing services are proposed to increase 6 percent a year.

Similarly, services for the elderly are among the "Cinderella" services identified to be substantially strengthened. An average annual growth rate of 3.2 percent is proposed for these activities. The document declares: "the main objective of services for elderly people is to help them remain in the community as long as possible."

The next year these policies were confirmed in a statement of the Government's national strategy for health and personal social services, "The Way Forward." It is recognized that adjustments in the "balance of care" towards greater support in the community would probably be "gradual and slow." It is also noted: "progress will vary from place to place depending on economic constraints, local choice and differences in the existing level of provision."

A subsequent DHHS policy statement in 1981, "Care In Action" maintains the essential thrusts of the earlier documents. Special concerns for the very elderly (over 85) are emphasized. The document urges personal responsibility for health and opportunities for prevention, while reaffirming the objective "to foster and develop community care for the main client groups, the elderly, mentally ill, mentally handicapped and disabled persons and children." It calls for further efforts to "strengthen the primary and community care services, together with neighborhood and voluntary support, to enable elderly people to live at home."

The 1981 statement also emphasizes "local initiatives, local decisions and local responsibility." Still, while the national department has "no monopoly of wisdom, . . . a National Health Service must also have regard to national policies and priorities." In light of the limited new resources,

> further progress cannot be rapid and will depend mainly on skilfull use of innovative approaches. . . . (Local) authorities will face conflicting pressures, and the need to expand and improve services for the growing number of

elderly people and the emphasis on care in the community are coupled with rapidly rising costs in some sectors of health and welfare services, particularly hospital services.

The commitment to strengthening community services is also set forth in a consultative document on "Care in the Community" issued by the DHSS in 1981. A report to Parliament the same year on elderly issues, "Growing Older," states: "the aim of the Government's policies is to enable elderly persons to live independent lives in their own homes wherever possible—which reflects what the majority themselves want." It also indicates: "providing adequate support and care for elderly people in all their varying personal circumstances is a matter which concerns—and should involve— the whole community, not just politicians and officials or charitable bodies. It is a responsibility which must be shared by everyone."

ORGANIZATION AND SCOPE OF SERVICES

In the following six sections, the organization and scope of home health services and related services in England are described. The primary health care team is discussed first, and then its principal members are considered separately. Other community health services, related social services and other pertinent community services are also reviewed briefly.

An extensive network of services is involved in maintaining individuals in their homes. A listing of 25 such services is presented in Table 1, along with their usual sponsors; this listing is based on a "Checklist of Services for Support in the Home" presented by A.A. Gatherer, a local medical officer (Shegog, 1981, pp. 55–67). Not only do the NHS and other parts of the National Government contribute critical support but so do local governmental authorities and private agencies. Health services are an essential part—but only a minor part– of the total system of support.

"The term 'community care' seems to mean very different things depending on the context in which it is used," notes the 1981 DHSS report on "Community Care." It is sometimes used as a description of existing services, e.g., community care

TABLE 1

SERVICES FOR SUPPORT IN THE HOME

Function	Service	Sponsor			
		NHS	Nat'l. Gov't.	Local Gov't.	Private Agency
Health	1 Primary health care team	X			
	2 General practitioner	X			
	3 District nurse	X			
	4 Health visitor	X			
	5 Other nursing services	X			
	6 Other health services	X			X
Income	7 Pensions		X		
	8 Special financial help		X		
	9 Cut-price schemes (e.g. transport, recreation)			X	X
Social	10 Social workers			X	
	11 Home helps			X	
	12 Day centers			X	X
	13 Elderly clubs			X	X
	14 Luncheon clubs			X	X
	15 Meals on Wheels			X	
	16 Aids to daily living	X		X	
	17 Domiciliary laundry	X		X	
Housing	18 Home maintenance			X	X
	19 Telephone			X	
	20 Home adaptation			X	
	21 Sheltered housing			X	X
	22 Warden schemes			X	X
	23 Residential homes			X	
Education	24 Adult education			X	X
	25 Library services			X	X

is those services provided outside institutions. In other cases, it is a statement of objectives, e.g., community care should enable an individual to remain in his own home rather than receiving long-term care in a hospital or residential home.

The attraction of community care, one analyst has pointed out (MacIntyre, 1977), is that it presents a way of resolving the humanitarian and organizational concerns in caring for the elderly. The former seeks to ameliorate the suffering which may accompany the aging process. The latter aims to limit the burden of dependency placed by the aged on society as a whole.

The network of supporting services is to meet twin chal-lenges—maintaining independence despite handicap, and ensuring help promptly when needed. Various services con-tribute to these objectives in different ways. As discussed below, ensuring that available services are organized and deployed in a coordinated and effective manner calls for a high degree of understanding and expertise.

Primary Health Care Teams

The primary health care team is the backbone of commu-nity health services. It is a "partnership of professionals" and ancillary staff working together to provide primary health care on a continuing basis to individuals in their homes and elsewhere in the community. The nucleus of the team is the GP, district nurse and health visitor.

Many others may also be members of a primary health care team. Commonly participating are practice nurses, reception-ists, midwives and social workers. A broader approach may also include other health care personnel, such a dentists, clini-cal psychologists, psychiatric nurses, pharmacists, occupa-tional therapists, and physiotherapists. Further, collaboration between the team and specialized medical consultants, such as geriatricians, may often be important. In concept, the team's composition is not fixed but rather is a response to the needs of the individuals being served.

While roots of the primary health care team may be found in the historic Dawson Report of 1920, the recent impetus dates from efforts in the 1960s to strengthen primary care. Teams expanded rapidly in areas where general medical ser-vices were largely delivered by GPs organized in groups and where the population was relatively stable. The Health Ser-vice and Public Health Act of 1968 specifically sanctioned community nurses to work in GPs' offices, health centers and clinics as well as patient's homes.

The 1976 Priorities statement strongly encourages the de-velopment of primary health care teams. Their purposes are defined as:

   a. to improve the preventive and curative services in the
      community,

b. to allow for the increased workload resulting from the greater number of old people, and
c. to reduce demands on acute hospital services.

The 1981 DHSS report on "The Primary Health Care Team" defines the team as "an interdependent group . . . who share a common purpose and responsibility, each member clearly understanding his or her own function and those of the other team members, so that they all pool skills and knowledge to provide an effective primary health care service."

To facilitate relationships among team members, "attachments to practice" have been developed. Under these arrangements, district nurses, health visitors and midwives work with one or more GPs on a continuing basis, obtaining some or all of their caseload from the GPs' lists. These approaches replace, in whole or in part, the deployment of nurses on a geographical (patch) basis. Often the nurses have office space and other support in the GPs' offices.

A 1980 survey of nurses working in the community by the Office of Population Censuses and Surveys (OPCS) found that over 80 percent of district nurses and health visitors were attached to GP practices. The percent of attached district nurses varied among health districts from 57 to 100 percent. Attachments tended to be higher in suburban, growth and retirement areas; they were lower in inner city and rural areas. About half of the district nurses and 60 percent of the health visitors were attached to one GP practice, usually involving a group of practitioners; most worked with six or less physicians.

The Chief Nurse Officer of the DHHS pointed out in a statement on "Nursing in Primary Health Care" in 1977, that:

> Experience has shown that where health visiting and district nursing staff have been attached to general practice and have developed cooperative patterns of working with each discipline providing its own specific skills, the quality of service to individual patients and families has improved. It has been possible to develop preventive and educative services as well as meeting the clinical needs of the practice population.

A number of important benefits have been achieved by effective teams. These include better casefinding, more complete and responsive care, better patient education, closer follow-up and improved compliance. Refinements in record-keeping have often contributed to these gains.

Attachments have often worked well when there are adequate premises, such as in group practices and health centers. They have sometimes been ineffective and impractical in cases of "single-handed" practices, especially in inner cities and isolated rural areas. As discussed below, problem areas have received serious attention in a number of recent studies.

Team approaches can help identify elderly persons and others in need of care. Analyses of GPs' lists in terms of age and sex can be the basis of focused casefinding and surveillance activities, though such efforts are reported to be not yet widespread. For example, a register of those "over-85-living-alone" has been suggested as a priority effort to encourage periodic visiting.

Teams have many different working arrangements, and relationships among members are varying and complex. Formal statements of duties have not been formally established. An analysis of team operations in the London area (Hughes & Robert, 1981, p. 11) points out: "the term 'team' is commonly used, easily understood, yet sufficiently ambiguous to allow all parties involved in the delivery of primary care to interpret and develop the idea differently while still believing that they are involved in the same enterprise." Different professional backgrounds and perspectives inevitably influence the attitudes and behavior of team members; while such differences add strength, they can also create tensions. Substantial effort is usually required to establish and maintain successful teams; in some cases, little effective teamwork has been achieved despite attachment arrangements (Hughes & Roberts, 1981, pp. 94–98).

Questions about the value of teams have been raised in recent years. In a few areas, nurses have been "detached." The Royal College of Nursing (1977) has criticized their "haphazard development," noting that "while attachment does bring together the diciplines involved in primary care, it does not of itself engender the team approach."

To address these concerns, a Joint Working Group on the

Primary Health Care Team was set up in 1978 by the Standing Medical Advisory Group and the Standing Nursing and Midwifery Advisory Committee. Their report, issued by the DHSS in May, 1981, identified a variety of obstacles to effective team operations. In some cases, large caseloads have confounded relationships. Further, pressures from different administrative systems are often experienced; GPs are independent practitioners with direct clinical responsibilities whereas nurses and some other team members are employees of local health authorities with diverse functions. Often there is inadequate understanding of the capabilities and concerns of different team personnel. As in other inter-disciplinary activities, issues of status, roles and leadership arise. Studies have pinpointed proper preparation and continuing communication as essential elements in affective team operations.

Other problems develop when the patients on GPs' lists are widely dispersed and where there a large number of persons not registered with a GP. These difficulties tend to be especially serious in inner city neighborhoods, such as inner London. The large number of "single-handed" practices in some of these areas provides further complication. Roberts (1982) has found that teams "scarcely exist" in parts of inner London. These problems have sometimes been met by combining attachment and geographical assignments, limiting GP practices to defined zones, reverting entirely to geographical deployment of nursing staffs, and focusing team efforts on nursing services.

The serious difficulties of providing services in inner cities have received special study. For example, the London Health Policy Consortium issued a report in 1981 on "Primary Health Care in Inner London." Among their many findings is the observation (p. 90) that: "with a large group of professionals operating in the same area there is bound to be an overlap of responsibilities and scope for changing the boundaries between different professions." They consider whether nurses might take on more responsibilities, allowing GPs to concentrate on more serious medical problems, and how patient counselling is best handled. They question if duties might be divided among GPs, nurses and social workers to achieve more efficiency. They urge further health services research to address these types of issues.

Still the important contribution of primary health care team receives widespread support. The 1981 DHSS report on "The Primary Health Care Team," for example, notes (p. 45):

> The problems of declining urban areas and the difficulties associated with providing effective primary health care services in such areas makes it very difficult for the team concept to work properly. . . . At the same time, however, the increased need for effective primary health care services makes the primary health care team all the more desirable. The strongest arguments both for and against the concept of the team have come from those responsible for providing primary health care in these areas

The report recommends additional resources for primary health care, including more adequate facilities, and urges steps to improve inter-personal relationships and team management.

The Royal Commission on the NHS concluded, in its 1979 report, that "the development so far of the primary health care team has been encouraging, but there is a continuing need to encourage closer working relationships among the professions who provide care in the community." The Commission identifies the provision of services in declining urban areas as the major challenge to community services and recommends more research into the methods of delivering primary care.

The Joint Working Group on Primary Health Care Teams (DHSS, 1981) also concluded that "the concept of the primary health care team is viable and should be promoted wherever possible." They proposed that where attachments are not feasible, other approaches to continuing collaboration among health workers be adopted. While they too recognize circumstances which make it difficult or impossible to provide primary health care on an integrated basis, such as certain inner-city neighborhoods, the report recommends (p. 50) extensions of primary health care teams to avoid

> the loss to the patient of the benefits of comprehensive and continuous care and a general reduction in personal fulfillment and satisfaction for the staff involved. At a

time when the advantages of providing care in the patient's home whenever possible are increasingly apparent, it is vital for primary health care services to be provided on a comprehensive and coordinated basis.

The 1980 OPCS survey of community nurses found that about 80 percent regarded themselves as primary care team members. A similar portion report good or very good contacts with GPs. Over 70 percent felt they had good or very good opportunities for discussions with clinicians.

Parallel to the development of multi-professional teams for the delivery of primary health care has been the establishment of similar teams for planning services in many local districts. These groups are concerned with the availability of services throughout the district, often with special focus on the needs of the elderly. They generally have a broad membership, including persons responsible for community services at the district health authority and representatives of GPs, the Family Practitioner Committee, and the Community Health Council as well as local government personnel concerned with social services and sometimes housing and education.

Planning teams advise the relevant district management teams and others and have no management responsibilities. In some cases, they have been able to develop an effective network of understanding and relationships and to help overcome problems due to diverse geographical boundaries. At their best, they have carried out important studies and exercised substantial influence on policy and operations (Shegog, 1981, p. 198). The potential roles of such planning teams in linking services have been increased by the additional centrifugal pressures resulting from the 1982 reorganization of the NHS.

General Medical Practitioners

There are about 23,000 GPs in England, approximately 5 per 10,000 population. There are two major differences in their practice patterns from those familiar in the U.S.: (1) patients usually see their GP first and do not normally have direct access to specialist medical consultants who work primarily in hospitals, and (2) GPs do not usually care for hospitalized patients.

Over 80 percent of GPs practice in partnerships of two or more physicians. Over two-thirds are in groups of three or more. About 17 percent work in some 700 health centers; this figure exceeds 20 percent when part-timers are included.

The average list of a GP includes about 2300 persons. It has been decreasing in recent years. (The British Medical Association recommends an average list of about 1700.) GPs select and reject registrants and, thus, can determine their list size and the extent of commitment to NHS work. GPs decide how they organize and conduct their practices, including partnership and staffing arrangements, what type of facilities they will have and when they will retire. In practice, few undertake much outside work.

GPs receive practice allowances and capitation payments from the NHS for persons registered with them. The capitation is higher for persons between 65 and 74 years of age and still higher for those 75 and older. The contract with the Family Practitioner Committee calls for the GP to provide all necessary and appropriate services within the scope of general practice to those registered with them, including referral to other health and social services.

GPs may obtain payment from the NHS for 70 percent of the costs of two staff members, either professional or clerical. Many employ "practice nurses" in their offices. About 1500 such nurses were reported in 1978.

General practice has been re-vitalized in England since the 1960s, somewhat similar to the changes in the U.S. . . . There has been increased emphasis on family practice in undergraduate medical education, more attention to postgraduate training, and establishment of a Royal College of General Practitioners. The number of GPs has been increasing about one percent a year, with the largest increases among female physicians and immigrant male physicians.

Continuity of care is one of the major benefits of a "robust system of general practice." Advantage in the care of the elderly can be substantial. A 1977 study of "Access to Primary Health Care" by the OPCS (1981, p. 53) found that 42 percent of the respondents had been registered with their present GP for 20 years or more or since birth; among those 65 years and older, the ratio was 60 percent.

Ideally GPs assume a comprehensive approach to the

physical, psychological and social aspects of patient care. An average consultation time of about five minutes, however, inevitably limits the scope of attention. Increasing attention to preventive care is being emphasized; GPs receive special "item for service" payments for certain such services, e.g., immunizations, cervical cancer examinations and antenatal care.

Most GPs contract to provide services 24 hours a day. In group practices, they usually cover for each other and may be on call one or two nights a week. Commercial services to provide night and weekend cover have become common in larger cities; concerns have been raised about the uses and quality of some of these arrangements, especially in London.

The distribution of GPs is controlled by the designation of "over-doctored" and "under-doctored" areas. In the former, which have average lists under 1900, contracts with new physicians are strictly controlled under the NHS. In the latter, which have average lists over 2500, incentives to develop new practices are offered. In London, serious concerns have developed about areas designated "over-doctored," largely because of short lists of elderly physicians. To address these issues, the Royal Commission on the NHS (1979) recommended improved retirement programs and arrangements for local health authorities to employ physicians and provide adequate premises in declining urban areas.

The 1977 OPCS survey of "Access to Primary Health Care" (1981, pp. 20-26) found that about three-quarters of the populations were within two miles of their GP; about 80 percent in urban areas and 50 percent in rural areas. Elderly persons are the most likely to have travel problems; elderly women had the most difficulty. About 30 percent of the population had four or more medical consultations during the previous year; this number increased to 33 percent for those 65 to 74 years of age and to 42 percent for those 75 and over.

Home visits during daytime hours had been requested from a GP by about 25 percent of the population during the previous year. For those 75 and over, home visits were requested by about 40 percent; four or more visits had been requested by 11 percent. About 10 percent of those requesting a home visit reported there had been an occasion when the GP had not come. Over 80 percent indicated it was easy to arrange such visits (OPCS, 1981, pp. 59–63).

Requests for home visits outside of normal office hours were reported by about 30 percent of the population during the previous five years. About 85 percent were successful in arranging such visits; 65 percent with their GP and 20 percent with another physician. Four of five of those who saw a doctor did so within two hours (OPCS, 1981, pp. 63–69).

Not all persons are registered with GPs, however. While accurate data on the unregistered is not available, studies in London have identified areas where 25 percent of the population was not registered. The London Health Policy Consortium study (1981) identified a number of causes: high population mobility, lack of interest, lack of knowledge, and inability to identify a willing GP. While Family Practitioner Committees are responsible for ensuring registration arrangements, this resource is not always known or used. A large proportion of those not registered are believed to be at high risk of illness, and many use hospital accident and emergency departments.

Some GPs make special provisions for the care of elderly registrants. They schedule off-peak office hours, and have "well elderly" clinics, emphasizing check-ups and preventive medicine. To encourage more efforts of this nature, there have been proposals that GPs be paid for additional "items of service" encouraging preventive care to the elderly and that demonstration projects on preventive practices be initiated, such as regular screening of those over 75 years of age.

About 15 percent of the average GP practice is elderly. This ratio varies widely, increasing greatly in retirement areas and some inner-city neighborhoods. While there has been a marked reduction in recent years in the frequency of home visits by physicians, some GPs are reported to continue to make regular home visits to their elderly registrants.

Specialized advice on the care of the elderly is available to GPs in most districts from consultants in geriatric medicine. In addition, some GPs are developing a "special interest" in geriatrics. It has been suggested (Shegog, 1981, p. 123) that a Diploma of Geriatric Medicine be available to GPs, similar to that offered in obstetrics and proposed for pediatrics.

District Nurses

District nurses, sometimes called home or domiciliary nurses, provide skilled nursing care and other support to persons living in the community. They are State Registered Nurses (SRN), who have had three years of basic training in a hospital and usually supplementary training in district nursing. They work as part of a district nursing team, which may also include a number of SRNs, State Enrolled Nurses (SEN), who have two years of basic training in a hospital, and nursing auxiliaries, who usually work in patients' homes.

About 13,700 district nurses were reported in 1979, about one per 3400 population. This group together with some 18,000 other primary care nurses, including health visitors, compose about 9 percent of English nurses. (A 1980 survey of U.S. registered nurses found that community health and school nurses account for about 9 percent of American nurses.)

The 1976 Priorities document noted that home nursing had been increasing about 6 percent a year and called for continuation of that rate of increase. It reiterated the staffing guideline, set in 1972, i.e., one district nurse per 2500-4000 population. The lower figure is for situations with a high proportion of elderly or disabled persons or extensive GP attachments. These services were viewed as especially important in the care of the elderly.

District nurse teams include about 17,000 members, a ratio of about 1:2700. In addition to district nurses, the teams include a few hundred SENs and about 3000 auxiliary staff (DHSS, Community Care, 1981, pp. 102–110). Staffs have increased 4-5 percent a year in recent years, somewhat less than the target rate set in 1976.

Training in district nursing involves at least six months specialized preparation in an educational institution. More than 70 percent of the SRNs employed as district nurses have received certificates. Specialized training became mandatory in September, 1981; training is to precede, rather than to accompany, practice. There may also be three months of supervised practice. (Training for SENs in district nursing lasts four months.) Local health authorities finance such training from their regular budgets in return for at least a year of service;

more centralized funding has been proposed in order to expand such training.

District nurses provide other services in addition to skilled nursing care in the home and clinic. They assess the needs of patients and families, supervise and lead other team members, monitor the quality of care, and arrange other support. In addition, they often advise patients on self care and educate family and other voluntary care-givers. Ideally, they have continuing and close familiarity with their clients and other community resources. Figure 1 illustrates the practice environment of district nurses (Royal College of Nursing, 1980).

District nurses are usually attached to GP practices as a member of the primary health care team. In other cases, they may be "aligned" or have other liaison arrangements with a number of GPs. As discussed previously, in some cases there have been problems in achieving effective teamwork. Other difficulties relate to excess travel, confidentiality of records, and problems in assuming new duties. Some nurses are reported to experience tensions due to dual loyalties to their primary health care team and district nursing management.

The recent sample survey of nurses working in the community (OPCS, 1982) provides information on the current characteristics and activities of these personnel. Table 2 summarizes major findings. It is especially noteworthy that district nurses devote about 90 percent of their patient care time to home visits and spend about 75 percent of their time in assisting elderly patients.

In 1979, district nurses provided care to about 70 of every 1000 persons in the population, an increase from 58 per 1000 in 1978. The average caseload was about 240 persons and the average length of a home visit was about 20 minutes. Over 40 percent of patients were first seen at their homes; this ratio increases to over 65 percent for the elderly. In some London districts, over 80 percent of the patient load is composed of elderly patients, most of whom are female (Poulton, 1977).

Arrangements for a district nurse to make a home visit may be made by a GP, hospital staff, social service worker, family and friends as well as by the nurse herself. The 1977 OPCS study of primary health care (1981, pp. 72–82) found that over 70 percent of the visits to the elderly were initiated by a GP, who provided instructions. The respondents (who were

FIGURE 1.

THE ENVIRONMENT IN WHICH DISTRICT NURSES WORK

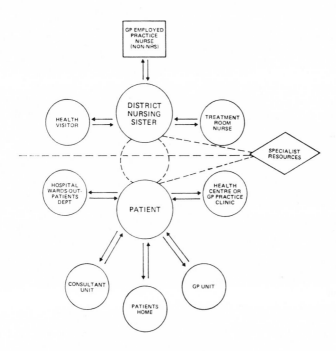

Source: Royal College of Nursing, Primary Health Care Nursing:
A Team Approach (Report of a working party of the Rcn
Society of Primary Health Care Nursing), published by
the Royal College of Nursing of the United Kingdom,
Henrietta Place, Cavendish Square, London W1M 0AB, 1980.

all consumers of care) reported that the most frequent services received from district nurses were changing dressings (43 percent), injections (26 percent), and medical checks (10 percent). Only two percent of those visited by a district nurse would have preferred to see a GP.

District nurses themselves indicated, in the 1980 OPCS

TABLE 2

FINDINGS FROM THE 1980 SURVEY
OF NURSES WORKING IN THE COMMUNITY

Characteristics/Activities	Percent of District Nurses	Percent of Health Visitors
Characteristics		
All community nurses	33	20
F.T.E. community nurses	35	25
Female	96	99
Full-time	82	83
Education		
Special certificate	72	99
Refresher courses	71	83
Management training	30	43
Working conditions		
Work base at home	61	6
Assistance with clerical work	15	57
Use of interview/treatment room	61	88
In community over five years	51	58
Attachment arrangement		
Some arrangement	83	89
Full attachment	47	37
Attachment plus patch	24	25
Serve all parts of GPs' areas	62	49
Work with one-two GP practices	66	79
Work with one-six GPs	65	77
Identify self as team member	84	77
GP contacts good/very good	80	71
Team meetings good/very good	39	42
See GPs daily	60	31
Alloction of working time		
Travel	24	16
Non-clinical activities	26	46
Patient care activities	48	35
Allocation of patient care time		
Home visits	89	56
Clinics	5	26
Serving elderly	74	9
Allocation of patient care work		
Technical assessments	2	14
Technical procedures	40	2
Other nursing care	38	3
Counseling and education	17	73

survey, that they devote about 40 percent of their patient care efforts to technical procedures (e.g., injections) and a similar portion to other nursing care. About 20 percent is spent on advisory activities, such as counseling and education. About 25 percent of their patients have physical handicaps, 15 percent cardiovascular problems and a similar percent skin problems, 8 percent diabetes, 5 percent mental handicaps, and 10 percent are receiving terminal care.

The district nurse respondents to the recent OPCS survey (1982) also indicated that they usually had good or very good knowledge of their areas (93 percent) and their patients (89 percent). A large portion (64 percent) felt they had good or very good knowledge of their patients' families. About 90 percent believed that the quality of care and 80 percent that the continuity of care were good or very good. About 70 percent were satisfied with their access to patients' records.

About 20 percent of elderly persons in England receive care during a year from a district nurse. This figure has increased from 15 percent in 1975 despite the increase of older persons. For every 1000 persons 65 years and over, there are about 4 community nurses who work primarily with the elderly (including district nurses, nurses with joint assignments, geriatric nurses and auxiliaries); the ratio varies from about 2 to over 6 among health districts (OPCS, 1982). This staffing level provides about 4.4 hours of community nursing services per week for every 100 elderly persons.

A study of district nursing services in 1973 (Ashley, 1977) found that 15 percent of the patients needed "high care," whereas 22 percent needed "intermediate care" and 63 percent "low care." In most cases, care was an alternative, rather than a supplement, to hospital care. A study in 1977 confirmed that about 20 percent of the patients receiving care at home were highly dependent.

Many district nurses report they feel over-burdened by the increasing responsibilities and pressures. Inner-city areas, especially inner London, present very difficult working and living conditions. As a result, there are high turnover and vacancy rates in some areas (Hughes, 1979; Hughes & Roberts, 1980).

The established national staffing guideline for district nurses, 1:2500-4000, is considered by many to require updating and revision in light of changes in both health care delivery practices and employment patterns. Increases in early discharges from hospitals, day surgery and clinic activities—as well as more elderly patients and more immigrants with language problems—require additional resources. On the other hand, decreases in working hours (from 40 to 37–1/2 hours a week) and increases in holidays and training courses have reduced available time. Other approaches have also been suggested, such as greater delegation to other nursing team members, especially for the care of early discharges and chronically sick patients. Others (Down, 1975) have argued that staffing norms should be related more directly to patients' needs, particularly dependency levels. The London Health Policy Consortium proposed, in 1981, that the staffing guidelines be increased 20 percent in recognition of high turnover, heavier workloads, and inexperienced staffs.

The utility of national staffing guidelines has also been questioned in view of the wide variations in local conditions and practices. Staffing ratios for district nurses varied among local areas in 1979 from 1:2200 to 1:5600; over three-quarters were below 1:4000 (DHSS, Primary Health Care Team, 1981). An analysis of staffing patterns in the London area concluded that they were related to historical practices, rather than to identified needs, potential efficiencies, or national guidelines (Hughes & Roberts, 1980).

The 1981 DHSS report on "Community Care" considered the value of national staffing guidelines and reached a positive, but cautious, conclusion (p. 51):

> Many guidelines have been set in isolation, rather than taking account of the complementary nature of some services. . . . (Still) they would seem to be helpful, if they are used with discretion. There is some evidence that (local) authorities consider them convenient, albeit imprecise, yardsticks for service planning. Interpreted sensibly, they may provide a useful barometer of under and over-provision which authorities need to probe in taking a strategic look at services. In the area of community-based services, they also serve as a fixed point in the local bargaining process.

The 1981 DHSS report on "The Primary Health Care Team" highlighted two other issues concerning community nursing services. It identified needs in certain local districts for 24-hour services to provide "out-of-hours" cover. It also noted uncertainties in the appropriate balance of skills on the community nursing team and proposed further review and research along these lines.

Concern for the slow development of community nursing resources has been expressed by many analysts and supporters. For example, a district nursing leader recently pointed out (Kratz, 1982): "District nurses can never refuse the admission of patients because the beds are never filled. They will give such care as will prevent a crisis developing but the quality of care they can give and their subsequent job satisfaction will fall." She urges greater efforts to document unmet needs, to increase understanding among physicians and social workers regarding appropriate referrals, and to expand innovative practices.

Other leaders have recommended that district nurses give more attention to health promotion and disease prevention activities. They believe these approaches are a natural and desirable extension of ongoing work in the home. More attention is being given to these topics in the restructured curriculum. About 60 percent of district nurses indicate (OPCS, 1982) that they would like to spend more time in counselling and health education.

About 45 percent of community nurses reported in the recent OPCS survey that there were needs for more care among elderly persons living alone. About 20 percent indicated other elderly persons also have serious unmet needs for services in the home. Approximately 15 percent identified persons with terminal illnesses as a priority problem needing additional services.

The 1981 DHSS policy statement, "Care in Action," calls again for more district nurses to strengthen primary care services. Their contribution to the implementation of the priority interest in extending care for the elderly at home is re-emphasized. The increasing need is dramatized by the fact that persons over 75 years of age receive more than three times as many services from district nurses as those between 65 and 74 years of age.

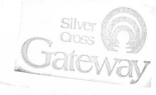

Health Visitors

Health visitors are concerned primarily with the promotion of health and the prevention of illness. Their development has roots in Florence Nightengale's concern for "nursing the well." Health visitors are SRNs with specialized training on the normal processes of growth and aging and family relationships. She is usually part of a health visiting team which may include other SRNs, SENs and nursing auxiliaries. Most of the work of health visitors has traditionally been focused on child health care, but more attention is being given to the elderly in many local districts. The recent OPCS survey (1982) found that overall health visitors spend about 10 percent of their patient care time serving elderly patients.

Health visitors visit persons and families on their own initiative in the absence of medical crises. They set their own schedule and priorities and initiate follow-up action on behalf of clients. They often visit households whose members have no other regular contact with the NHS and thereby identify unknown physical, mental and other problems. Health visitors are also concerned with the early detection of illness, surveillance of high-risk groups, and health teaching.

Training in health visiting involves 12 months specialized preparation in an educational institution. Such training has been mandatory since 1946, and centralized funding was begun in 1981. Increasing attention is being given in the curriculum to the behavioral sciences and the community environment.

The 1976 DHSS Priorities statement proposed that health visiting services also be expanded six percent a year. It reiterated the staffing guideline, set in 1956, for one health visitor per 3000–4300 population. The lower figure is for areas with highly developed systems of attachment or with large immigrant populations.

There were about 8100 health visitors in England in 1979, a ratio of about 1:5700. The ratio varied among local districts from 1:2900 to 1:7300 (DHSS The Primary Health Care Team, 1981). Health visiting teams also include an additional 1300 SENs and auxiliary staffs, producing a team ratio of 1:4900 (DHSS, Community Care, 1981). Recent growth in health visiting staffing has been three to five percent a year, a rate below the 1976 target.

Shortages of health visiting staff are common. This problem is especially serious in urban areas. As a result, staffs often include a relatively large number of newly trained nurses (Hughes, 1979).

About seven percent of the elderly receive health visiting services during a year. Elderly persons are typically visited two or three times a year.

Because health visitors initiate and arrange their own work, schedules and priorities tend to vary widely (Clark, 1981). While there are routine systems for learning about new births, there is no similar approach for identifying needs of the elderly. About 20 percent of the elderly persons visited by health visitors are referred by GPs and 10 percent by hospitals. A study of home visits to the elderly by health visitors (Clark, 1976) found that the most frequent issues addressed were arrangements for social services, care of specific illnesses, diet, general health, and adjustment to illness.

Health visitors are also commonly attached to GP practices. Because the tradition and training of health visitors emphasize independent work and responsibilities, many have experienced difficulties in developing effective team relationships (Hughes & Roberts, 1981). Further efforts to extend mutual understanding and cooperation have often been encouraged. It has been suggested that the increasing interests of many GPs in prevention may further complicate some relationships. Many health visitors work on a geographical basis, even when they also have attachment arrangements, in order to reach the unregistered and to maintain their intimate knowledge of the community.

In some places, health visitors have undertaken surveys of the elderly, using age registers from GPs' practices and screening activities. These efforts are aimed at identifying unknown illnesses, increasing awareness of needs and identifying gaps in services, especially among persons over 70 years of age. These activities produce referrals to both medical and social services.

Modification of the national staffing guidelines for health visitors has also been recommended. Many believe that updating is appropriate in view of changing workloads and working hours. In addition, some have urged that further delegation of tasks to less skilled staffs working under supervision be considered. More efforts to match work plans to high risk conditions and more vulnerable groups, such as the elderly, have also been urged; the training and perspectives of health visitors regarding human growth and development, it has been noted, provide a very relevant framework for additional services to the elderly (Kinnaird, 1981).

Geriatric health visitors and geriatric visitors have been employed in some local districts to concentrate efforts on the needs of the elderly. These types of personnel are not yet widely distributed; they compose only about one percent of all community nurses. The recent OPCS survey (1982) identified these types of personnel in only half of the surveyed districts; over 60 percent of the total were in two districts. The number and distribution of these workers may increase in view of the increasing number and needs of the very elderly.

Other Community Health Services

A considerable number of other community health services help maintain individuals in their own homes. These resources supplement the work of primary health care teams, providing specialized services. Ideally, they are all integrated into comprehensive local networks, even though most are part of related hospital services.

Community psychiatric nurses have been increasing in recent years (Parnell, 1978). There are about 2000 such nurses, who provide care to an estimated 50-60,000 persons. About 30 percent of their time is reported to be devoted to the elderly (OPCS, 1982). Most patients have been discharged from hospitals, but there are also referrals directly from the community. Advice and support are given to primary health care teams; some work out of GPs' premises and health centers, although they are managed as part of the hospital psychiatric services. It is estimated there are 7–10 community psychiatric nurses as an average per health district, ranging from 2 to 20.

Day hospitals provide care to the geriatric and psychogeriatric patients. They are extensions of the related hospital services. Places in these facilities have expanded relatively rapidly in recent years. (These services are closely related to the day centers, which are discussed below; in some cases, overlap of services and activities has been reported.)

Geriatric day hospitals began in the 1950s and have steadily expanded (Brockelhurst, 1981). There are about 300 in Great Britain, proving about one place per 1000 elderly. (The DHSS guideline is 2:1000 elderly.) About 20 percent of the elderly population received care in a day hospital in 1978, an increase from 16 percent in 1975 (DHSS, Community Care, 1981). The availability of transportation, and the cost thereof, are important aspects of this service.

Similarly, places in psychiatric day hospitals have expanded since the 1940s. There are about .3 places per 1000 population in 1978. This ratio is about half the national guideline, .65:1000.

Dental care is arranged on the basis of "courses of treatment." Dental practitioners contract independently with the NHS; while they may have private patients, NHS and private treatment of individual patients may not be undertaken concurrently. About 25 percent of the elderly with some natural teeth report regular dental visits (OPCS, 1981). Where necessary, dentists may visit elderly patients in their homes to assess needs and may in special cases provide treatment there.

Most vision tests, over 80 percent, are given by opticians, who also contract with the NHS. Over 80 percent of the elderly report a sight test within the last five years; about 50 percent within the last two years (OPCS, 1981). While domiciliary visits are rare, they can be arranged; extension of such services for the disabled elderly has been proposed.

Community physiotherapy services are a recent development. They are directed at maintaining the mobility of the elderly and other disabled patients and at instructing families in the management of frail and disabled old persons. About three quarters of the local health districts are reported to have such services, which are linked to related hospital services.

Occupational therapists employed by the NHS, who are based in hospitals, are making an increasing number of home visits. Their work includes assessments, treatments and instructions to the family. In some districts, speech therapists also provide services to patients in their homes.

Chiropody services can help prevent immobility among the elderly and others. About 80 percent of such patients are age 65 and older. Over three-quarters of the services of chiropodists are provided in the community, and one quarter are given in the home. There is about one chiropodist per 5000 elderly. While the number of chiropodists has been declining, the number of foot care assistants has been increasing. The 1976 DHSS Priorities statement calls for an annual growth rate of three percent for these services, but shortages of personnel make it unlikely this objective will be reached soon.

A number of other community health services are available in some local districts. For example, in some localities, dietitians are assigned to community activities. Nursing aids are sometimes made available to those requiring such help, and hearing and vision aids are also supplied in some cases.

Other Community Services

A variety of other community services make critical contributions in enabling the elderly and others to live in their own homes. Some are financed by local government and others by private and voluntary agencies. Payment is required for most of these services, with sliding scales for those less able to pay.

Social services are provided largely through social services departments of local government. In 1978, there were about 22,000 social workers, about .5 per 1000 population. While social service staffs working in the community are assigned on a geographic basis, many are part of the primary health care teams in GPs' practices and health centers. Between 15 and 20 percent of their time, it is estimated, is spent with the elderly (DHSS, Community Care, 1981).

Home helps from social services departments provide many essential services in homes, especially for elderly persons living alone. Every local social services agency is required, under a 1968 law, to provide an "adequate" home help service. These workers assist in such domestic activities as cooking, cleaning and shopping; usually they make two or three visits a week to a household and have an average caseload of 7–8 persons. Daily visits and 24-hour coverage may be provided to help meet emergencies and after hospital discharge. Problems in ensuring coverage early in the morning, late at night and on weekends are reported from some areas (Davis & Challis, 1980).

In 1979, there were about 90,000 home helps working an average half-time, thus making available about 45,000 full-time equivalents. In addition, there are about 2000 full-time organizers. This is a staffing ratio of about 1:1000 population or 7:1000 elderly. (The 1976 DHSS Priorities statement set a national guideline of 12:1000 elderly.) About 90 percent of their services are given to persons 65 years of age and older; about 60 percent to those 75 and over. Over half their clients are seriously physically handicapped. In 1979, about 95 of every 1000 elderly persons received assistance from home helps during the year; the rate was 175 per 1000 for those 75 and over (DHSS, Community Care, 1981).

Innovative approaches to providing home help services are being developed in some areas, particularly for more vulnerable elderly patients. In some districts, care assistants and care attendants are providing a combination of social and nursing care. In others, volunteer "helpers" are extending services at relatively modest costs; young elderly persons are an important part of these groups (Davis & Challis, 1980).

Day centers have expanded rapidly in the last few years. About half these places are for the elderly. In 1980, there were almost 3 places per 1000 elderly, compared to about 1.5 places per 1000 in 1975. In addition, there is about 1 day care place per 1000 elderly in residential homes for non-residents. Some centers are full-time and others part-time. Most participants attend once or twice a week; few attend every day. The 1976 DHSS Priorities document calls for 3–4 places per 1000 elderly, a target that appears to have been substantially achieved (DHSS, Community Care, 1981).

Local authorities also assist the elderly and others to meet housing needs. In some cases, such assistance enables individuals to continue to reside in their own homes. In other cases, residential homes and sheltered housing are made available. Only a very brief summary is possible here concerning the substantial efforts made along these lines.

Structural changes to existing homes make it feasible for many older persons to remain at home. These activities include widening doorways, installing handrails and lifts, and arranging needed equipment, such as telephones. Alarm call systems in some areas facilitate prompt assistance in emergencies; radio and automatic alarm equipment and mobile support teams are being tested in a few localities (Shegog, 1981, p. 15).

Sheltered housing brings together a group of elderly persons in congregated and self-furnished small apartments. There may be a common meeting room, along with a recreational program and noonday meals. A warden usually provides or arranges emergency assistance and may also provide other support, such as help in shopping, property maintenance, and referrals to community agencies. Wardens are usually middle-aged women with backgrounds similar to the residents; there have been some concerns about a tendency of wardens to assume excessive responsibilities (Hermann, 1980). These arrangements provide protective and social support as well as housing.

Residential homes have been described as the "keystone of provision" of community services for the elderly (Davis & Challis, 1980). The 1976 DHHS Priorities statement points out: "in general a greater need for residential accommodation is likely in those localities with a large number of old people living alone in unsatisfactory accommodations, remote from relatives, friends, shops, and other facilities. . . . Provision of sheltered housing may reduce this need."

Residential homes are managed by local social services departments as well as by private and voluntary agencies. The private facilities are inspected by public agencies and usually receive some public funding. Typically four to six persons share a room, but some homes have single rooms. About 23 places were available for every 1000 elderly in 1976 (DHSS, Community Care, 1981); the national guideline set forth in the 1976 DHSS Priorities statement was at least 25 per 1000 elderly.

About 95 percent of the permanent residents in residential homes are 65 years of age and older; 80 percent are 75 or older. The average age of admissions has been rising and is near 82. In some cases, patients stay for short periods, usually to meet emergencies and to provide respite for families and other caregivers. Every resident is required to pay a charge, at least a minimum related to social security benefits, but most facilities are subsidized by local authorities. Some units have limited nursing staffing and have been compared to certain nursing homes in the U.S.

Domiciliary meal services assist the frail elderly who can not participate in luncheon clubs. A common arrangement is two meals a week. In some cases, such as recent hospital discharges, full meal service may be provided for a limited period. In 1980 about 120 meals were served each week per 1000 elderly persons; the 1976 DHHS Priorities guidance was 200 meals weekly per 1000 elderly. About two-thirds are provided in recipients' homes. About half are given by public agencies and half by private groups (DHSS, Community Care, 1981).

A number of other services are made available in certain localities. For example, special transportation may help elderly persons reach day centers, day hospitals and other destinations. Some libraries arrange services to the housebound as well as to day centers and residential homes. Adult education programs and recreational activities are designed in some communities to meet interests of the elderly.

LESSONS FROM THE ENGLISH EXPERIENCES

From the review of efforts in England to maintain the elderly in their homes to the maximum extent feasible, I have identified seven lessons that appear worthy of special consideration. Many—perhaps all—of these points are familiar to most health care students and practitioners. Still, further discussion of these issues may help reenforce past learning and encourage additional analyses of factors important in providing home health services and related services to the elderly in their homes.

The seven lessons may be summaried as follows:

1. Home health care services and other community services are intimately related,
2. Voluntary services are essential to home health care,
3. Changes in community services and hospital services strongly affect each other,
4. Close linkages to psychiatric services are important,
5. Special educational and training efforts are needed,
6. Cost analyses are complex and often uncertain, and
7. Progress is usually slow and difficult.

Each of these points is reviewed in turn in the second part of this analysis.

THE INTIMATE RELATIONSHIPS
BETWEEN HOME HEALTH AND OTHER SERVICES

Health care services have tended to be separated from social services and other community services in England, as in the U.S. Professional, organization and funding differences all contribute to divisions. However, efforts to meet the increasing needs of the elderly have reemphasized the many critical inter-relationships; coordination and even integration of services is receiving more attention. The Royal College of Nursing (1977, p.13) has pointed out: "Many of the problems of older persons are multi-factor and often relate to social problems; as age increases, the dividing line between 'medico' and 'socio' becomes more blurred."

The work of home helps in England in the delivery of care in the home is an impressive example of the inter-relationships. These workers, who are employed by social services departments, make it possible for many primary health care teams to maintain additional persons at home. They often are able to make the earliest assessment of changing health conditions and to alert health care professionals and others to developing needs.

Similarly, the availability of adequate housing arrangements frequently determines whether medical and nursing care can be provided at home or whether hospitalization must be arranged or continued. An effective alarm system can make it feasible for elderly persons to live at home while providing assurance that needed health services will be called promptly in emergencies. Relatively minor structural changes and special equipment can make the difference between living at home and entering an institution.

The availability of adequate income may be the most important single determinant of an individual's capacity to live independently and well. Retirement ages in England are generally 60 for women and 50 for men. National retirement pensions are augmented by supplementary benefits, tax credits and other support, such as attendance allowances for severely disabled persons and exemptions from prescription charges.

"Individuals require a package of services suited to their needs if they are to be cared for in the community. No one community-based service is likely to be able to shoulder the burden of providing an alternative to long-term hospital or residential care," observed the DHSS in the 1981 report on "Community Care." Similarly, a recent analysis of aging issues sponsored by the Nuffield Provincial Hospital Trust (Shegog, 1981) concludes: "A successful policy for care of the old depends upon a combination of housing, food, care, and social contact suitable to each individual. A break at any point in the chain nullifies the value of the rest." This review also points out (pp. 63, 66):

> It is in the nature of problems in the older person that they are seldom simple; even if the trigger event is clearly social or physical, there is a rapid evolution of a mixed bag of secondary problems. . . . (Still), steady co-ordinated assistance in daily living as independence moves in fits and starts toward more dependency will probably ensure that a majority (of older persons) remain at home for most of the time in their final years.

A "balance of care" approach, which is being initiated in some districts, illustrates the inter-relationships of services. Elderly persons are classified according to levels of need, and alternative packages of care are designed to meet assessed needs. Table 3 indicates five possible ways of caring for one type of patient; nursing services, home helps, meals-on-wheels and day care may be combined in different mixes to maintain the individual at home or care may be provided in a residential home or hospital. The alternative packages present guidelines for potential trade-offs and changing resources.

A variety of mechanisms aim at better collaboration and coordination among the different services. At the delivery level, the efforts of primary health care teams are fundamental. At administrative levels, communication and common efforts are facilitated by board representation, joint consultation committees, joint finance projects, and staff coordination schemes; a brief review of some of these approaches may indicate the scope and diversity of the efforts along these lines.

Joint consultation committees are composed of representatives of the NHS and local governmental agencies. They were

TABLE 3

ALTERNATE PACKAGES OF CARE
FOR ONE CATEGORY OF ELDERLY

Resource	Unit	Packages				
		1	2	3	4	5
Own home	days per week	7	7	7		
Home nurse	visits per week	3	2.5	1.5		
Home help	hours per week	16	12	6.5		
Meals on wheels	number per week	3	1.5			
Day hospital	days per week		1.5			
Day center	days per week			4		
Residential home	days per week				7	
Hospital	days per week					7

established after the NHS reorganization in 1974 to overcome some of the divisive aspects of that action. The committees, which are advisory in purpose, may undertake joint studies and oversee joint finance projects. Many are reported to have encountered difficulties due to differences in the attitudes and expectations of members, inadequate preparation and staff support, and lack of influence and resources (Flynn, 1980). More forceful approaches have been recommended, such as the development of joint strategies, plans and agreements; local actions to strengthen collaborative activities can be encouraged and assisted, it has been pointed out (Shegog, 1981, p. 23), by more effective coordination at the national level.

Joint finance projects are financed from NHS funds to aid selected social service activities which can relieve pressures on the health services. Local public agencies and voluntary agencies sponsored by them may receive funds for operating or capital expenditures. Project plans must provide for the transfer of continuing financial support to local sources (usually after seven years). The limited period of NHS support has been a constraint on joint efforts in some cases, and their scope has been limited by the exclusion of housing and education services. NHS funds for these types of projects increased fourfold between 1976 and 1980; about 40 percent have been for the elderly, such as extensions of home helps, care assistants and night sitting services, and improvements in residential homes.

Staff coordination activities include joint planning teams with personnel from local health and social service agencies. Specialists in community medicine are members of social service management teams in some localities, and health service liaison officers from social services departments are sometimes appointed to health service planning teams. To strengthen these efforts, additional inter-authority and inter-professional staff groups have been recommended (Shegog, 1981, p.201) with clearer responsibilities for analyzing needs, developing related plans and policies, and formulating specific implementation steps; the increasing needs of the elderly are seen as a stimulus and priority for such efforts.

Effective collaboration is not easily achieved, however. The Royal Commission on the NHS noted (1981, p.261) that "health and local authorities have different functions; while health is the preoccupation of health authorities, it is only one of several competing responsibilities of local authorities." For example, the development of housing to enable the elderly to live in the community may compete with needs for new schools. These strains are more intense in times of economic difficulties, a common contemporary condition.

The 1981 DHSS consultative document on "Care in the Community" identified (p. 1) needs for "more social service provision . . . both to keep up with the rising number of very elderly people and to provide for those being cared for in hospitals who might be better cared for in the community." It analyzes a number of methods of financing such additional activities, including (a) extension of joint finance projects using NHS funds, (b) annual capitation payments, and (c) pooling responsibilities and funds for specific client groups. The report emphasizes the importance of offering incentives to both health and local government authorities in order to develop more services in settings most appropriate to the needs of individual clients.

The intimate relationship among health and other community services is aptly summarized in a recent analysis of aging issues (Shegog, 1981, p. 189):

The health of the elderly is inseparable from their social care and accommodation. A health problem presents itself as a social problem; a social problem as a health problem. In the tasks of prevention, caring, curing and rehabilitation, health facilities, social provision, and mode of accommodation are interdependent and there are wide, gray areas where it is hardly possible to distinguish one from the other. It follows that the provision of health and social services and special accommodation must be closely inter-related if the results are to reach expectation.

THE ESSENTIAL CONTRIBUTIONS OF PRIVATE AND VOLUNTARY SERVICES

"Care *in* the community must increasingly mean care *by* the community." In this statement, the DHSS report on "Growing Older" (1981) highlights the critical roles of family members, friends, neighbors and voluntary agencies in maximizing opportunities for the elderly to live at home. Most of elderly living at home depend on such help for essential support; it is estimated that about 40 percent receive help from relatives (Pinker, 1980). The 1981 DHSS report notes that proportionally more older persons are currently being aided by their families than at the beginning of the century and emphasizes that: "It is the role of public authorities to sustain and, where necessary, develop—but never to displace—such support and care."

The 1981 DHSS study of "Community Care" concludes (p. 54) that only the availability and commitment of family members and other voluntary support makes it feasible for many persons to remain at home. "Informal care" is often especially important for those requiring intensive support. Family and friends are often the main "primary care team."

Much of the work of organized public and private agencies supports and supplements informal care networks of relatives, friends and neighbors. Primary health care team members are often most valuable in aiding family and other informal caregivers who, in turn, support an elderly person. Some community services, such as home helps, night sitting, day centers and short-term admissions to residential homes, are frequently as important for the relief they afford informal caregivers as for the direct support to elderly individuals.

Voluntary activities are very diverse in nature and sponsorship. The 1981 DHSS study of "Community Care" classifies them into five categories: informal carers, neighborhood care groups, mutual aid and self-help groups (e.g., stroke clubs), individual volunteers, and formally organized agencies. Voluntary efforts in the personal social services are estimated to exceed the number of hours of service provided by paid staffs.

The amount of voluntary services, some analysts anticipate, will increase with reductions in working hours and years. However, these gains may be largely offset by such factors as increases in employed women, geographic mobility and smaller houses. One observer (Pinker, 1980) has cautioned, for example; "It is neither accurate nor fair to assume that women will have the willingness and the capacity to provide the bulk of (needed) services." Further, caring for the larger number of very elderly is likely to require more skill, attention and time.

The development of effective relationships among public and voluntary programs requires special care and resources. Joint planning, liaison officers and service coordinators facilitate coordination in some communities. Both health authorities and social services agencies work with voluntary groups in most localities, sometimes providing them modest fiscal support. The 1981 DHSS consultative document, "Care in the Community" points out: "It is easier to harness the energy and resources of the voluntary sector if people are in the community."

Volunteers also help provide information to the elderly and others through Citizen Advice Bureaus and similar activities. Guidance and counselling is often needed to help individuals find their way to and through the bewildering maze of pertinent agencies and services. These efforts can also help improve communications and referrals among public and private agencies.

Another mechanism of voluntary participation and influence is the Community Health Councils, whose purpose is to represent the views of consumers in the NHS. Since 1974 every local health district has had such a body, usually including 20 to 30 members, at least one-third of whom are appointed by voluntary organizations. Many carry out surveys of local services and participate on NHS planning teams. In some cases there has been confusion and controversy about their roles, similar to those experienced by some consumer bodies in the U.S.

The Royal College of Nursing (1977, p. 25) has summarized the recent history and current conditions of voluntary activities in the following terms:

> The relationship with the voluntary services has deteriorated because in the early years of the (NHS) emphasis was placed "on getting away from charity." Moreover, organized labor has sometimes been hostile, fearing that paid staff would be ousted by "free labor." These fears are unfounded and there is need to rethink attitudes to the voluntary services. Firstly, the need for help with older people in the community will be insatiable; this demand cannot be met by professionals nor is it appropriate that it should be. What many older persons need more than a professional service is someone to take an interest in them.

THE DYNAMIC INTERACTIONS
BETWEEN COMMUNITY AND HOSPITAL SERVICES

Changes in hospital services frequently have a direct impact on demands for home health and other community services. Similarly, the availability of home health and related services affects arrangements for admitting and discharging patients from hospitals. These interactions and complex and dynamic in England, as elsewhere.

Reductions in the length of hospitals stays, which have been occurring in England, as in the U.S., increase pressures for follow-up care in the community. Likewise, expansions of ambulatory surgery have generated additional demands for home care. The impact is greatest on district nurses and, in many cases, family care-givers.

On the other hand, inadequacies in available community services can result in avoidable hospital admissions and extended stays. "Bed-blocking" has been a serious problem in many cases for both acute and long-stay hospitals. Further, hospitals are often burdened with tests and treatments that could be handled in the community. However, the potential impact of changes is uncertain; the 1981 DHSS report on "Community Care" notes (p. 68):

> Some elderly people are at present inappropriately placed in hospital beds, given the lack of any more suitable alternative, (but) equally some residents in local authority homes should be in the hospital. It is therefore necessary to think of patterns of care for the elderly as involving movements in both directions.

The care of the elderly in England is influenced importantly by the development of the medical speciality of geriatrics since the 1940s (Brockelhurst, 1975). A 1981 DHSS study of the care of the elderly hospital patients points out (p. 2):

> "From its origins as a 'last resource" service for elderly patients who did not respond to treatment in the traditional specialities, geriatric medicine developed into a medical sub-speciality concerned with the clinical, preventive, remedial and social aspects of health and disease in elderly patients.

While these specialists concentrate on the treatment and rehabilitation of hospitalized patients, they also work with and provide advice to primary health care teams and other community services. Hospital geriatric services have been described as "the crucial underpinning" to community services for the elderly (Shegog, 1981, p. 145).

Geriatricians are a shortage medical specialty, however. In 1979, there were about 400 consultants in geriatric medicine and 300 others in training positions. Additional incentives to increase recruitment have been proposed. About 40 percent of the consultants are foreign born (compared to 15 percent of all medical consultants) and the proportion is even higher for those in training. At least one geriatric consultant per 10,000 elderly has been recommended but the current supply is less than half that ratio. In addition to providing clinical and advisory services, geriatricians often act as a pressure group on behalf of better care for the elderly.

Geriatricians direct geriatric hospitals and departments of geriatric medicine in general hospitals. These facilities may include three types of beds: acute care beds, rehabilitation wards, and long-stay or continuing care wards. About 75 percent of the patients in geriatric facilities are 75 years of age or older. The overall average length of stay is about 80 days, but it has been declining steadily.

The DHSS guideline, set in 1962, calls for 10 geriatric beds per 1000 elderly. Of this number, 3 are to be in the main District General Hospital (DGH) for assessment and acute treatment, 2 are for active rehabilitation and 5 are for longer-stay patients, preferably in small local hospitals where patients are near families and friends. In 1982, there was about 8.2 geriatric beds per 1000 elderly, but inadequate numbers were in DGHs. Ideally, multi-disciplinary geriatric teams in the DGH are "centers of expertise," providing advice and assistance to other hospital services and those caring for the elderly in the community.

Most hospitalized elderly patients in England are admitted to non-geriatric hospital services. Other departments treat over 75 percent of all non-psychiatric inpatients who are 65 years and older. About 40 percent of the patients in general medicine and surgery are elderly. Studies have identified needs for added training of the personnel staffing these units concerning the multiple medical and social problems of the elderly.

Communications between hospital and community services is a concern in some situations. A 1978 study of such relationships found "few structured systems." The Royal Commission on the NHS observed (1979, p. 43):

> There is frequent criticism of communications across the hospital/community boundary; hospital staffs complain of patients being referred to them without adequate documentation and GPs complain of patients being discharged to their care without warning or information. While there are well established conventions between doctors for handling over a patient from hospital to the

community, or vice versa, the development of such conventions between nursing staffs has been slow.

Similarly, the London Health Policy Consortium's study of health care in inner London (1981, p.80) reported: "Sometimes GPs and other primary care workers are not informed of the discharge and there are problems of referral to local authority social services such as home helps and meals on wheels." These problems can be especially serious for elderly persons living alone.

Liaison nurses have been appointed in many hospitals to coordinate admission and discharge procedures between the hospital and community services and to facilitate the flow of information. Many are former district nurses or health visitors and others are social workers. Their activities supplement the direct channels that sometimes exist between community nurses and hospital ward sisters and the efforts of social workers and some volunteers. In some cases, geriatric liaison nurses have been employed to focus on the needs of the elderly.

Increased participation of GPs in the care of hospitalized elderly patients has been proposed as a means of enhancing professional relationships and continuity of care (London Health Policy Consortium, 1981, p. 84). Their work can be especially important in local community hospitals, where as many as two-thirds of the patients may be elderly and where stays may continue for extended periods. The expansion and upgrading of these facilities in many communities has been delayed because of fiscal constraints.

The development of nursing homes within the NHS is a recent innovation. Some analysts have urged action along these lines as a priority (Pinker, 1980); there appears to be sensitivity to problems experienced in many U.S. nursing homes. Three experimental efforts were undertaken in 1982 to study whether this approach can provide a better alternative than current arrangements in hospitals and residential homes. The new nursing homes are under nursing direction, include 25–30 beds and aim to meet the emotional, psychological and spiritual needs of the patients in a domestic-oriented environment.

THE INCREASING IMPORTANCE
OF LINKAGES WITH PSYCHIATRIC SERVICES

"Perhaps the most serious single problem for the future is going to be the management of the increasing number of patients suffering from senile dementia," a British geriatrics expert has commented (Brockelhurst, 1975, p. 40). The incidence of this problem among the elderly is estimated at about 10 percent and is expected to rise, especially among the increasing number over 75 years of age. The Royal Commission on the NHS noted (1979, p. 58): "The major problem of mental illness is now the dementia of old people, and it is therefore impossible to plan services for the old and the mentally ill separately."

The intimate interrelationship of problems creating disabilities among the very elderly are emphasized in the DHSS report on "Growing Older" (1981, p. 50). "From the age of 75, medical, social and psychological problems become increasingly common. A close link between physical and mental conditions present special problems in diagnosis; mental confusion may be caused by physical illness, and mental disturbance may complicate physical illness and delay recovery."

The implications of these conditions for home health care are very great. For example, the 1981 DHSS study of "Community Care" points out (p. 38):

> Most of those suffering from dementia live alone or are looked after by their families and friends; for every person in long-term residential care, five are at home. A high level of provision of domiciliary support—particularly home helps, meals-on-wheels, day care facilities and community psychiatric nurses, are necessary if those less severely affected by dementia are to be maintained in the community and not impose an intolerable strain on friends and relatives. For some sufferers, such support is not enough and they need to be in residential homes. For others, short-stay admissions in residential homes or hospital can provide sufficient relief to rela-

tives and friends to enable them to continue for some time to be the main supporters.

As discussed above, the number of community psychiatric nurses has been increasing. These nurses work in the community with patients, families, primary health care teams and others. In some districts, their efforts are almost entirely devoted to the care of elderly patients.

Psychiatrists with a special interest in the elderly are also expanding. These specialists not only provide direct care but also advise GPs, heads of residential homes and others. They also work with specialists in geriatrics and other medical specialties. A short-term objective is at least one psychiatrist with a special interest in the elderly in each health district. The Royal College of Psychiatrists has recommended one consultant session for every 2000 elderly (1000 in teaching districts) but this ratio has not yet been approached in most places.

Day hospitals, day centers and residential homes are other community resources of special importance in helping those with mental illness. Ideally, these services are part of an integrated program, along with hospital, home health and other community services. The expansion of facilities in smaller community hospitals to provide more of the care for the elderly severely mentally infirm patients has been planned so that patients are closer to families and friends and community support is enhanced.

Overlapping services are a concern in view of the similarities in the "model" services for the elderly and the elderly mentally ill. Duplication may not only be costly but also may confuse families and GPs. Separate services have developed in some areas due to such factors as the impact of dementia upon elderly persons and their care-givers, the distinct professional identities of medicine and psychiatry, and the risk that those afflicted with dementia may be overlooked in light of the greater number of physically handicapped elderly. To address these concerns, it has been proposed (Shegog, 1981, p. 18) that mechanisms for joint assessment and review be established in each health district, including the participation of GPs, geriatricians, psychiatrists, nurses, social workers, housing, and other services.

NEEDS FOR SPECIAL EDUCATIONAL AND TRAINING ACTIVITIES

Three types of needs for education and training activities have been identified for special attention:

1. to make multi-disciplinary teams more effective,
2. to enhance knowledge and skills concerning the elderly,
3. to strengthen inter-agency planning and collaboration.

While these issues should all be addressed, at least in part, during the basic preparation of health professionals, and other affected disciplines, existing gaps make supplementary efforts desirable and necessary.

As indicated in the discussion of primary health care teams, their operations have often been complicated and impaired by inadequate understanding among team members of the capabilities and viewpoints of their colleagues. Further education is one approach towards overcoming these problems. The Royal Commission on the NHS noted (1979, pp. 267–268) that:

> post-reorganization experience shows that effective collaboration requires that those involved should have appropriate training. . . . More emphasis (is needed) on the education and continuing education of health and social work professionals in the importance of inter-professional collaboration.

Similarly, the 1981 DHSS report, "The Primary Health Care Team" found (pp. 24, 52):

> the need for more multi-disciplinary training, and training in the specific communication and inter-personal skills required for working in a team, to be included in nurses' and doctors' professional training. . . . The concept of teamwork . . . (should) be actively promoted through continued training at all levels, particularly within a multi-disciplinary framework.

While some joint training programs have been implemented along these lines, the small size of these activities has meant that relatively few have had opportunities to participate.

Understanding of the needs of the elderly is important not only for those specializing in the care of the aged but for all health care and social service workers. Initiatives to this end are underway. For example, geriatric issues have been introduced into the basic curriculum for district nurses and health visitors, including instruction and practical training. Opportunities for education in geriatric medicine are being made available to an increasing number of medical students; the Royal College of General Practitioners and the British Geriatrics Society recently recommended such training for all undergraduates and reenforcement during postgraduate years. In-service training of staffs of public and private agencies has also been expanded. Still there are questions whether existing efforts are equal to the challenges presented by the increasing needs of the elderly.

The third subject requiring special attention is the advancement of planning and management capabilities. The complex nature of community service programs calls for a high degree of expertise to ensure effective arrangements for bringing together the many related agencies and resources. A recent review (Shegog, 1981, p. 11) concluded that while

> a number of excellent instances of management initiatives in establishing joint teams working between the NHS, social service and other departments (had been identified), such achievements are often due to experience and training in "corporate planning" which, however, are lacking in many managers at all levels. . . . In addition to specialist skills, senior managers at every level need professional-presented analyses of policy and project innovations to equip them for the difficult environment in which they operate. Education of this nature ought also to be used deliberately as a communication bridge between different levels of management and different services.

Further attention to these issues are likely in the future.

THE COMPLEXITIES AND UNCERTAINTIES OF COST ANALYSES

The 1981 DHSS study of "Community Care" included a review of 25 "cost-effectiveness" research studies (pp. 12–21, 73–75). It was found that none were comprehensive or complete. They failed to measure all the resources and costs of caring for individuals at home and elsewhere in the community and were limited in duration. In many cases not all of the related public outlays were included; commonly private costs were entirely excluded. Substantial methodological difficulties were usually encountered, particularly in considering different levels of dependency.

However, a number of pertinent points are presented in the review and analysis:

1. Community-based care often depends on the services of informal care-givers (e.g., families, friends and neighbors), but the costs of their services are very difficult to document, especially the loss of employment opportunities;
2. The cost-effectiveness of community care appears to depend often on not putting a financial value on the contributions of informal care-givers, who may in fact experience considerable financial, social and emotional burdens;
3. The higher the level of dependency, the more services are usually required and the greater the costs;
4. Those who live alone tend to receive more services;
5. Community-based packages of care are not always the least expensive and most effective, especially for persons living alone;
6. Reported economies may be due to the absence of necessary or adequate services;
7. "Borderline" cases (i.e., those at the margin of home, residential and hospital care) tend to require the most intensive services; and
8. Individuals not receiving any services are usually less dependent and would generally utilize less expensive services.

The costs of alternative "packages of care" for the elderly were analyzed in a few special studies in an effort to identify more cost-effective approaches. The results of an analysis carried out by the DHSS in Devon in 1978 are presented in Table 4. The study considered the costs of NHS and public personal social service costs for persons then being served; 32 categories of dependency were analyzed, taking into account physical and mental conditions and social circumstances. Unmet needs and private services were not included. Resources and fiscal costs of different packages of services which had been identified by local professionals were calculated. The

TABLE 4

POSSIBLE PATTERNS OF CARE IN THE EXETER HEALTH DISTRICT;
RESOURCES AND COSTS PER 1000 ELDERLY PERSONS

Resource	Unit	Estimated Resources for			National Norm
		Maximum Effective- ness[1]	Minimum Cost[2]	Compro- mise[3]	
District nurse	full-time	1.0	1.0	.9	1.7[4]
Home help	full-time	18.1	13.7	17.9	12.0
Meals	per week	112.0	114.0	110.0	200.0
Day hospital					
geriatric	places	.6	.2	.7	2.0
psychiatric	places	.7	1.9	.4	2.0-3.0
Day center	places	2.0			
Residential					
home	places	7.6	16.7	8.6	25.0
Long-stay beds	beds	3.3	1.7	2.8	5.0
Mentally infirm					
beds	beds	4.3	.5	3.9	2.5-3.0
Estimated costs					
pounds[5]	thousand	118.0	82.0	111.0	144.0
NHS	percentage	55.1	35.4	53.2	56.3
Social services	percentage	44.9	64.6	46.8	43.7

Footnotes:
1. First preference of professional advisory team
2. The least expensive package of care
3. The least expensive of the preferred packages of care
4. Assumes about 60 percent of time is given to caring for the elderly
5. Based on 1978 local costs and is limited to public expenditures for NHS and social services

analysis included a "maximum effectiveness" package, a "minimum cost" package and a "compromise" package which attempted to balance cost and effectiveness. In addition, the estimated resource requirements were compared with national staffing guidelines.

As indicated in Table 4, the "compromise" package depends upon substantial services in the home. The "minimum" cost package involves more care in residential homes. The comparisons with national norms suggest that some guidelines do not adequately consider the relationships of individual services to the total array of potential services. The analysis of costs between the NHS and social services points to a need for greater growth in the latter, especially home help and similar services.

THE SLOW PACE OF PROGRESS
IN DEVELOPING COMMUNITY SERVICES

Despite the repeated statements of national policy in favor of more rapid development of services in the home and community, especially for the elderly, progress has been slow. While agreement in concept may be widespread, implementation in practice is difficult. For example, target rates for expanding community nursing services have not been achieved although the demands on these services has been expanding. A nursing leader (Hockey, 1978) has written: "an example of contradiction is the emphasis on community care as a national and local priority without the resources which could make such an emphasis a practical reality." In England, as in the U.S., national policies and guidelines are subject to various interests and interpretations among local and regional bodies and groups.

The rate of growth of home health and other community services has been slowed by overall constraints on available funds, existing commitments and practices, and intense competition for funds. Difficulties in the general economy have severely limited the amount of new resources available to the NHS and local agencies. Powerful pressures on behalf of hospital services and staffs have continued and even increased, making it very difficult to close institutions or particular services and to transfer resources from inpatient to community care.

Manpower constraints have also limited the growth of community services. Recruitment and training of district nurses and health visitors have not been adequate to achieve staffing targets. Home helps and nursing auxiliaries draw heavily upon the same supply of middle-aged women, whose numbers are decreasing and whose opportunities for other positions are increasing. Health services research efforts have yet to clarify uncertainties concerning the most appropriate mix of professional and supporting staffs.

However, there have been noteworthy increases in recent years in the numbers and percentages of elderly persons receiving certain community services. District nursing, home helps, meals-on-wheels and day care, for example, have expanded. Nonetheless, the large majority of the elderly living at home do not receive any organized services and few receive intensive services; district nurses serve less than 20 percent and home helps less than 10 percent during a year. It has been estimated that about 20 percent of the elderly have needs for organized services on a long-term basis.

The 1981 DHSS study of "Community Care" found (p. 3) "little identifiable shift in the balance of care for those elderly persons on the margin between institutional and community-based care." The report notes (pp. 30, 67):

> It may be questionable whether the present community-based services can and should reduce the proportion of elderly people in long-term hospitals and residential care. Particularly intensive and relatively expensive services may be needed (for this group). . . . The level of certain domiciliary services and the frequency with which people attend day hospitals and day centers, for example, do not suggest that in general sufficiently intensive packages of care are being offered, particularly to those with no informal or neighborhood network to support them.

> It may well be that other objectives of community services are considered more important, for example, improving

the quality of life for people for whom there is no question of institutional care, providing short-term treatment in the care of community nurses, or crisis intervention in the case of social workers. . . . The risk is that diffusion of effort will result in no one objective being achieved and the least efficient deployment of resources.

Home care and community services have been sometimes supported, at least rhetorically, without careful attention to their strengths and shortcomings. Pinker points out (1980, p. 274) that: "both governmental and non-governmental authorities have tended in the past to emphasize what care in the community can accomplish and to give less attention to what it cannot do."

Providing adequate community services in inner cities, such as London, has been especially difficult. The combined impact of widespread social deprivation, high population mobility and limited primary health care resources has convinced some analysts that adequate community care in these situations may be a "pipedream" (Roberts, 1982). The 1981 report of the London Health Policy Consortium proposed a series of major actions to address these problems, urging that "the voice of community services should be strengthened and be given a more effective hearing in the structure of management . . ."

It is evident that greater resources will be required in the community to meet the increasing needs and expectations of the elderly. The Royal Commission on the NHS observed (1979, p. 70):

Services for the elderly will make increasing demands on health and local authorities for the rest of this century. We are concerned that without greater shift of resources than are yet evident neither health nor local authority services will be able to cope with the immense burden these demands will impose. Inevitably the community as a whole will have to share the responsibility and cost of caring for the elderly at home with appropriate support from the health and personal social services. . . . In the NHS the burden of caring for infirm old people will fall mainly on nurses, and efforts must be made to encourage them in undertaking this work.

Despite the difficulties that have been encountered, the policy and commitment in England for home care and related community services remain strong. While the pace of change has been constrained by many conditions and forces, the general direction of development has been maintained. For example, the consultative document, "Care in the Community" indicates (1981, p. 1):

> "a great deal has already been done to enable more people to be cared for outside hospitals, but more could be done if resources of money and manpower were available. In the longer term, a further shift in the balance of resources from hospital to community services is desirable. . . . Most people who need long-term care can and should be looked after in the community. That is what most of them want for themselves and what those responsible for their care believe to be best.

The resolution of these issues depends in free societies upon the values and decisions of the public as a whole concerning the uses of the nation's wealth. The report on "Growing Older" asserts (DHSS, 1981, p. 2): "no society can call itself civilised if it treats its older generation with lack of consideration," while recognizing that "ultimately, the quality of life of elderly people, especially the very old and frail, rests on the attitudes and perceptions of those younger than themselves."

REFERENCES

Abel-Smith, B. *A history of the nursing profession.* London: Heinemann, 1960.

Ashley, J. Community care: Continuing or alternative care? *Royal Society of Health Journal,* 97–3, June, 1977, 127–130.

Brockelhurst, *J.C. Geriatric care in advanced societies.* Baltimore: University Park Press, 1975.

Brockelhurst, J.C. & Tucker, J.S. *Progress in geriatric care.* London: King's Fund Centre, 1981.

Clark, M.J. The role of the health visitor. *Journal of Advanced Nursing,* January, 1976, 25–36.

Clark, J. *What do health visitors do? A review of the research, 1960–1980.* London: Royal College of Nursing, 1981.

Davis, B. & Challis, D. Experimenting with new roles in domiciliary service: The Kent community care project. *The Gerontologist,* 20–3, Part 1, June, 1980, 288–299.

Department of Health and Human Services. *Health-United States,* 1981. Hyattsville, Maryland: DHHS Publication No. (PHS) 82–1232, 1981.

Department of Health and Social Security. *Care in action.* London: Her Majesty's Stationery Office, 1981.

Department of Health and Social Security. *Care in the community, a consultative document on moving resources in England.* London: Department of Health and Social Security, 1981.

Department of Health and Social Security. *Growing older.* London: Her Majesty's Stationery Office, 1981.

Department of Health and Social Security. *Health and personal social services statistics for England, 1978.* London: Her Majesty's Stationery Office, 1980.

Department of Health and Social Security. *Nurse manpower-maintaining the balance.* London: Her Majesty's Stationery Office, 1982.

Department of Health and Social Security. *Nursing in primary health care.* London: Department of Health and Social Security, 1977.

Department of Health and Social Security. *Priorities for health and personal social services in England, a consultative document.* London: Her Majesty's Stationery Office, 1976.

Department of Health and Social Security. *Report of a study of the acute hospital sector.* London: Department of Health and Social Security, 1981.

Department of Health and Social Security. *Report of a study on community care.* London: Department of Health and Social Security, 1981.

Department of Health and Social Security. *Report of a study on the respective roles of the general acute and geriatric sectors in the care of the elderly hospital patient.* London: Department of Health and Social Security, 1981.

Department of Health and Social Security. *The primary health care team.* London: Department of Health and Social Security, 1981.

Department of Health and Social Security. *The way forward.* London: Her Majesty's Stationery Office, 1977.

Down, J. & Smith, A.H. The deployment of home nurses. *British Journal of Preventive and Social Medicine,* 1975, 29, 53–57.

Flynn, M. Coordination of social and health care for the elderly. *The Gerontologist,* 20–3, Part I, June, 1980, 300–307.

Hermann, L. Sheltered housing for the elderly: The role of the British warden. *The Gerontologist,* 20–3, Part I, June, 1980, 318–329.

Hockey, L. District nursing today—the obstacles and opportunities. *Nursing Mirror,* 147–20, November 16, 1978, 58–60.

Hughes, J. and other. Nurses in the community: A manpower study. *Journal of Epidemiology and Community Health,* 1979, 33, 262–269.

Hughes, J. & Roberts, J.A. *Nurses managers' views of community nursing services.* London: London School of Hygiene and Tropical Medicine, 1981.

Hughes, J. & Roberts, J.A. *Problems in the development of London's community nursing services, in London's health services in the 80s,* edited by M. McCarthy. London: KF Project Paper, 25–3, April, 1980.

Jarman, B. Medical problems in inner London. *Journal of the Royal College of General Practitioners,* 1978, 28, 598–602.

Kane, R.L. & Kane, R.A. *Long-term care in six countries.* Bethesda, Maryland: Fogarty International Center Proceedings No. 33, NIH Publication No. 80–1207, 1980.

Kinnaird, J. & others. *Provision of care for the elderly.* London: Churchill Livingstone, 1981.

Kratz, C.R. *Community nursing—prescription for excellence.* Nursing Times, April 21, 1982, 676–682.

London Health Policy Consortium. *Primary health care in inner London, report of a study group.* London, May, 1981.

MacIntyre, S. *Old age as a social problem, in R. Dingwall and others, Health care and health knowledge.* London: Croom Helm, 1977.

Merry, E. & Irven, I. *District nursing.* London: Bailliere Tindall & Cox, 1960.

Office of Population Censuses and Surveys. *Access to primary health care.* London: Her Majesty's Stationery Office, 1981.

Office of Population Censuses and Surveys. *Nurses working in the community.* London: Her Majesty's Stationery Office, 1982.

Parnell, J.W. *Community psychiatric nurses.* London: Queen's Nursing Institute, 1978.

Pinker, R. Facing up to the eighties: Health and welfare needs of the British elderly. *The Gerontologist,* 20–3, Part I, June, 1980, 273–283.

Poulton, K.R. *Community nursing service of Wandsworth and East Merton teaching district.* London: St. George's Hospital, 1977.

Roberts, J. *Community care in London—A pipe dream?* London: London School of Hygiene and Tropical Medicine, 1982.

Royal College of General Practitioners. *Survey of primary care in London.* London: Royal College of General Practitioners, 1981.

Royal College of Nursing. *Evidence to the Royal Commission on the National Health Service.* London: Whitefriars Press Ltd., 1977.

Royal College of Nursing. *Primary health care nursing, a team approach.* London: Royal College of Nursing, 1980.

Royal Commission on the National Health Service. *Report.* London: Her Majesty's Stationery Office, 1979.

Shegog, R.F.A. *The impending crisis of old age: A challenge to ingenuity.* London: Oxford University Press, 1981.

Development of
Innovative Health Services
for the Frail Elderly:
A Comparison of Programs
in Edinburgh, Scotland,
and Rochester, New York

William H. Barker, MD

ABSTRACT. This paper delineates a model of health services for the elderly in industrialized societies and examines innovative developments in these services in recent years in Edinburgh, Scotland and Rochester, NY. Emphasis of innovations in the former has been upon early intervention in health problems of the frail elderly in the home and avoidance of hospitalization ("preventive geriatrics"). The focus in the latter has been largely upon improving efficiency and appropriateness of placement of elderly persons who require long term care. These experiences reflect the distinctive organization and financing of health services in the UK and the US as well as the exemplary efforts of professional leaders in identifying and addressing unmet needs of frail elderly persons in the respective communities studied. Opportunities for each society to benefit from the other's experience are discussed.

William H. Barker is Associate Professor in the Department of Preventive, Family and Rehabilitation Medicine, University of Rochester School of Medicine, Rochester, NY 14642.

This work was supported in part by a travel-study fellowship awarded to the author by the World Health Organization during the academic year 1982–83.

An early version of this paper was presented at the Annual Meeting of the American Public Health Association, Montreal, Canada, November 1982 and to the Scottish Branch of the British Geriatrics Society, Dundee, Scotland, March 1983.

The author would like to acknowledge Professor James Williamson and colleagues at the University of Edinburgh and Drs. Robert Berg, T. Franklin Williams and James Zimmer at the University of Rochester for their valued contribution to my appreciation of the developments reviewed in this article.

INTRODUCTION

The demographic imperative of aging populations with attendant increasing prevalence of chronic disease and disability is posing a challenge to the health services of all industrialized societies (Grundy, 1983). While the nature of health and health-related problems of the elderly in contemporary industrialized societies appear to be quite similar (Shanas, Townsend, Wedderburn, Friis, Milhoj and Stehouver, 1968), these problems are being addressed through a variety of health service innovations in different societies (Brocklehurst, 1975). Comparisons of such developments between one's own society and another affords an opportunity to identify significant differences as well as similarities of approach and to assess potential adaptations from each other's experience. The occasion of a sabbatical year based in the Department of Geriatric Medicine at the University of Edinburgh (Scotland) afforded an opportunity to closely observe and review development of innovative health services for the elderly in that community and to contrast these with developments in Rochester (New York), with which the author has worked for a number of years. Both communities have had unusually strong and sustained involvement in such health service innovation, hence their experiences may be viewed as at the forefront in their respective societies. The strikingly different orientations of innovation, the one emphasizing early identification and intervention in health problems, preferably in the patient's home (preventive geriatrics), the other emphasizing optimal classification and placement of chronically disabled patients with skilled nursing needs (long-term care), raises interesting questions to be discussed at the conclusion of the paper.

BACKGROUND

Settings

The two settings are broadly comparable in geopolitical, demographic and social parameters as shown in Exhibit 1. The land masses of the Lothian region and Monroe County, the political jurisdictions within which Edinburgh and Roch-

EXHIBIT I

SELECTED SIMILARITIES BETWEEN THE SETTINGS
OF EDINBURGH AND ROCHESTER

CHARACTERISTICS	(EDINBURGH) LOTHIAN REGION	(ROCHESTER) MONROE COUNTY
SIZE	670 sq. mi.	750 sq. mi.
GEOPOLITICAL COMPOSITION	Metropolitan area with many contiguous villages and surrounding rural areas	
POPULATION (1980)		
TOTAL	748,603	702,223
% $\geq$ 65	14.3	11.0
% $\geq$ 75	5.4	3.4
SOCIO-ECONOMIC CHARACTERISTICS	Relatively high income and employment and relatively little heavy industry	

ester are situated, both approximate 700 square miles, each consists of a single major city surrounded by contiguous villages and rural areas, and the populations are approximately three-quarters of a million. Proportions of elderly are somewhat higher in the Lothian area. Finally, both metropolitan areas are characterized by relatively high incomes and relatively little heavy industry, and both include one major academic medical center.

Health Care Systems

In contrast to the broadly similar geographic and social profiles of Edinburgh and Rochester, the financing, organization and planning of health services in their respective societies is strikingly different. The British National Health Service (with its counterpart Scottish Home and Health Department), has financed and set policy for development of comprehensive health services since its inception in 1948. As such, a single public budget finances all components of personal health services in the society. Principle planning and management functions are carried out by area health authorities, such as the Lothian Health Board, which cover population catchments of less than one to several million persons. Medical and nursing professions working through their professional societies or their institutional affiliations, play an active role in developing and implementing health service innovations in concert with the health authority within the area in which they practice.*

Personal health services in the United States are financed through a variety of public and private third party payors as well as by patients out-of-pocket. The predominant mode is fee for service and third party payors reimburse services selectively rather than comprehensively. Acute hospital care and long-term institutional care have been the dominant services covered by third party payors, while rehabilitation and home health services have been less well covered, hence less well developed. Regional planning and development of services has been encouraged by state and national government, but has accomplished little in most parts of the country. New

---

*For current discussion of health planning and decision-making in Great Britain, see Klein, R. *The Politics of the National Health Service.* London: Longman, 1983.

York State and the Rochester-Monroe County region in particular represent an exception, having a tradition of active community involvement in evaluation and controlling the development of the most costly resource, acute hospital beds, and more recently nursing home beds.

Health Services for Elderly Model

In comparing development of health services for the frail elderly, I have chosen to use the simple model in Figure 1 which envisions three principal situations in which the elderly person may be recipient of health services: in the home, in a general hospital or in a chronic care facility. Health services for the elderly are provided to varying degrees at all three of these loci in both the United Kingdom and United States and for that matter in virtually all industrialized societies. The question of interest is to define how the services function at each point in the spectrum, and in particular to determine which part of the spectrum of services has commanded the greatest attention in development of innovations in the two communities under study and why.

Briefly to define the dynamics of the model, one may start on the far right, where in fact the development of geriatric medicine originated, with frail elderly people housed in chronic facilities. The role of services at this point is largely a passive one of assigning patients to appropriate settings to provide for their level of dependency. This practice is commonly labelled "long-term care," as on the model. On the far left of the figure is care at home in the community. With the objective of maintaining the individual's highest degree of social, physical and mental independence as well as avoiding unnecessary admission to hospital or chronic institution, this part of the spectrum has aptly been labelled "preventive geriatrics," a term coined in Scotland (Anderson, 1974; Williamson, 1970).

The middle component of the model comprises the general hospital with its potential roles of providing rehabilitative care and often, unintentionally social care, as well as acute care for elderly patients. To the extent that it emphasizes rehabilitation, hence reduction of unnecessary dependency, the general hospital serves as part of the process of "preventive geriat-

FIGURE 1

HEALTH SERVICES FOR THE FRAIL ELDERLY

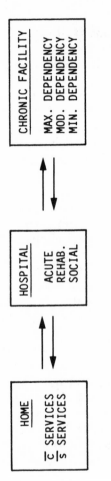

rics." If the emphasis in hospital is confined to acute care, persons with disability are classified as social disposition problems and the hospital assumes, albeit inappropriately and unwillingly, a long-term care role.

Having established this basic frame of reference, the balance of the paper will first briefly examine the essential elements of the model currently found in Edinburgh and Rochester; second, summarize landmark surveys of health care needs of the elderly conducted in both Edinburgh and Rochester in the early 1960s; third, review a selected series of specific initiatives to meet problems identified in the surveys in the two settings; and lastly, discuss lessons to be drawn from the rather different orientations of the two communities in identifying and addressing health care needs of their frail elderly.

OBSERVATIONS

Spectrum of Services, Edinburgh and Rochester

The essential elements of services in the two settings are summarized in Exhibit 2. Certain features are particularly noteworthy. First with respect to care of persons living at home, enrollment of virtually everyone with a general practitioner is an essential fact of life in Edinburgh as in all of the U.K. Furthermore community nurses (health visitors and district nurses) are commonly attached to general practice surgeries or health centers. In a recent survey of a representative sample of general practitioners in the Lothian area, over 75% reported such attachments of community health nurses (Barker, 1984). Domiciliary occupational therapy, meals-on-wheels and home helps for short-term and long-term management of patients in their homes are available from sub-area offices of the Department of Social Work. Under these circumstances nursing as well as social support services may potentially be easily coordinated with primary medical care for a defined group of patients. By contrast in Rochester and throughout the U.S. primary medical care may be provided by family doctors, office or hospital-based specialists or by house officers working in hospital outpatient or emergency depart-

EXHIBIT 2

HEALTH SERVICES FOR THE FRAIL ELDERY
EDINBURGH AND ROCHESTER (N.Y.)

	HOME	HOSPITAL	CHRONIC FACILITIES
EDINBURGH	GENERAL PRACTITIONER VISITING NURSE HOME HELPS OCCUPATIONAL THERAPY	ACUTE BEDS GERIATRIC UNIT ASSESS. & REHAB. DAY HOSPITAL	LONGSTAY HOSPITAL GERIATRIC PSYCHIATRIC RESIDENTIAL SHELTERED HSNG

———————— GERIATRICIANS ————————

	HOME	HOSPITAL	CHRONIC FACILITIES
ROCHESTER	"PRIMARY" M.D. VISITING NURSE HEALTH AIDES	ACUTE BEDS EXTENDED CARE	SKILLED NURSING HEALTH-RELATED PSYCH. INSTIT. CONGREGATE HSNG.

ments. Visiting nurses employed by private or public agencies are available for limited tasks, largely restricted to post-hospital care; rarely are they attached to physicians' practices. With limited exception (see ACCESS below), there is virtually no equivalent to the well-developed home help or domiciliary occupational health services found in the U.K.

In the general hospital sector, while an array of geriatric assessment and rehabilitation inpatient services as well as day hospital, are now widely provided in Edinburgh as elsewhere in the UK (Barker, 1983), in Rochester and throughout the U.S. hospitals are largely restricted to providing short-term acute medical and surgical care. Some hospitals provide a limited number of "extended care" beds for post-acute convalescence, but such beds are rarely used for geriatric assessment and rehabilitation as practiced in the U.K.

The types of chronic care facilities found in the two communities are broadly comparable. The US skilled nursing facility and intermediate care facility are analogous in level of patient dependency to the longstay hospital and residential accommodation, respectively. Longstay psychiatric institutions and sheltered housing are provided to limited degrees by public authorities in both communities.

Finally, the development of the specialty of geriatric medicine and attendant establishment of hospital-based geriatric medicine units throughout the country is a uniquely British institution (Brocklehurst, 1975; Barker, 1983). With direct responsibility for geriatric inpatient services and day hospitals and liaison with other inpatient services, primary medical care and social work services within a defined catchment area, the consultant in geriatric medicine is uniquely situated to effect coordinated development and use of services by elderly persons.

Health Service Innovations, Edinburgh

A widely cited survey of unmet health needs of elderly patients at home conducted in Edinburgh by Williamson and colleagues (1964) in the early 1960s was one of the first of several surveys in Scotland which focused attention on development of preventive health services for the elderly. This study, the essentials of which are summarized in Exhibit 3, concluded that early recognition and management of such

EXHIBIT 3

"OLD PEOPLE AT HOME: THEIR UNREPORTED NEEDS"

(Summary of Williamson, et. al., 1964)

PROBLEM
ELDERLY OFTEN HOSPITALIZED IN ADVANCED STAGE OF
DISABILITY; MUCH PREVENTABLE BY TIMELY INTERVENTION

PURPOSE
DETERMINE HOW WELL ELDERLY PATIENT NEEDS KNOWN TO GENERAL
PRACTITIONER

SURVEY
RANDOM SAMPLE OF PATIENTS $\geq$ 65 Y/O IN 3 GENERAL
PRACTICES IN LOTHIAN REGION

ASSESSMENT BY GERIATRICIAN, PSYCHIATRIST,
SOCIAL WORKER

FINDINGS
AVERAGE OF 3.35 DISABILITIES PER PERSON;
1.96 UNKNOWN TO GENERAL PRACTITIONER

RECOMMENDATIONS
DEVELOPMENT OF STRATEGIES FOR MORE EFFECTIVELY
IDENTIFYING AND ATTENDING TO HEALTH NEEDS OF
ELDERLY PATIENTS AT HOME

problems as depression, gait difficulties and incontinence among elderly persons living at home could reduce unnecessary decline in health and admission to hospital. A series of health service innovations all of which reflect a "preventive geriatric" orientation have been undertaken in Edinburgh in the ensuing years in response to this issue. A selection of these as listed in Figure 2 will be briefly reviewed.

As an initial follow-up to the 1964 survey, Williamson and colleagues (1966), worked with several general practices in Edinburgh to establish an early diagnostic service for elderly patients, staffed by health visitors (community nurses). "High risk" elderly patients, e.g., persons over age 75, living alone, recently bereaved or discharged from hospital, were selected from the general practice lists and invited to receive an assessment for unmet health problems. Among 300 consecutive patients, significant health impairments were detected in two-thirds, and recommendations leading to improved functioning were provided to approximately one fourth. The authors recommended that such services should be widely adopted through the offices of health visitors attached to general practices (Lowther, MacLeod, and Williamson, 1970).

A second anticipatory strategy, prompt home visiting to elderly patients referred by GPs for hospital admission, has been emphasized by the University of Edinburgh Department of Geriatric Medicine since its inception in 1976. This practice is intended to assure early intervention to prevent unnecessary decline in health in frail elderly persons as well as to assess the potential for the patient to be cared for at home instead of in hospital. In a series of 209 consecutive home visits by geriatricians, one or more potentially remediable social, nursing or medical problems were detected in the majority and solutions to problems by interventions other than hospital admission were achieved in 59% of instances. These included referral to day hospital for diagnostic assessment or rehabilitation, recommendations of a variety of changes in medical or social management at home and arranging future "holiday" relief for caretakers who were approaching exhaustion (Arcand and Williamson, 1981).

In a more recent initiative, the Department of Geriatric Medicine has developed a scheme of short-term augmented home care aimed at elderly patients who experience sudden

FIGURE 2

HEALTH SERVICES FOR THE FRAIL ELDERLY
SELECTED INNOVATIONS - EDINBURGH

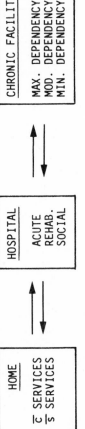

HOME
c̄ SERVICES
s̄ SERVICES

HOSPITAL
ACUTE
REHAB.
SOCIAL

CHRONIC FACILITY
MAX. DEPENDENCY
MOD. DEPENDENCY
MIN. DEPENDENCY

PREVENTIVE
GERIATRICS

LONG TERM
CARE

1. MONITORING HIGH RISK ELDERLY IN GENERAL PRACTICE

2. PROMPT HOME VISITS BY GERIATRICIANS TO G.P. REFERRALS

3. AUGMENTED HOME CARE SCHEME FOR ACUTE ILLNESS

4. GERIATRIC CONSULTATION ON ACUTE MEDICAL SERVICES

78

acute decline in health which traditionally cannot be managed at home and requires admission to hospital. Preliminary analysis of a series of hospitalized patients indicated that up to a third might be effectively treated at home by their general practitioner if short-term intensive nursing and/or social support services were available in the home. In a pilot study 37 acutely ill patients who were treated at home with augmented support services, rather than being hospitalized, were found to recover function in terms of Activities of Daily Living more rapidly than a comparable group who were hospitalized and with no untoward consequences (Currie et al., 1980). The scheme was deemed practical and acceptable and is currently being further evaluated in a controlled trial in Edinburgh under funding from the Scottish Home and Health Department.

A final innovation to be noted is the system of routine geriatric consultation on acute medical and surgical inpatient services, begun in Edinburgh in the late 1970s and subsequently widely emulated in Great Britain and abroad. This represents a response to the problem of "bed-blocking" by hospitalized elderly patients who following care of their acute problem remain excessively long in hospital for want of attention to rehabilitation and effective discharge planning. Through addressing these particular needs of elderly patients early in their hospitalization, the geriatric consultation service reduced mean lengths of stay for members of both sexes. This was most dramatic for women, falling from 25 to 16 days among all over age 65 and from 50 to 19 days for those over 85 years old. These changes were primarily achieved through returning patients to the community with appropriate support services rather than expediting placement in long-term care institutions (Burley, Currie, Smith and Williamson, 1979).

Health Service Innovations, Rochester

A landmark and again widely cited survey of health care needs of the elderly conducted by Berg et al. (1970) in 1964, was one of the first among a series of health service planning studies in the Rochester area which drew attention to the need to improve services for the long-term care patient. The study, summarized in Exhibit 4, focused particularly upon the

EXHIBIT 4

"ASSESSING THE HEALTH CARE NEEDS OF THE ELDERLY"

(Summary of Berg et al., 1970)

PROBLEM
NEED FOR RELIABLE DATA ON HEALTH CARE NEEDS OF
ELDERLY TO GUIDE DEVELOPMENT OF EFFECTIVE PROGRAMS

PURPOSE
ASSESS EXISTING FACILILTIES FOR CARE OF AGED
AND DEVELOP RATIONAL PLAN FOR FUTURE SERVICES

SURVEY
SYSTEMATIC SAMPLE OF NON-INSTITUTIONALIZED AND
INSTITUTIONALIZED PERSONS $\geq$ 65 Y/O IN MONORE CO.

ASSESSMENT BY GENERAL INTERNIST AND COMMUNITY NURSE

FINDINGS
47.1% OF INSTITUTIONALIZED ELDERLY INAPPROPRIATELY
PLACED, USUALLY RECEIVING TOO HIGH LEVEL OF CARE

RECOMMENDATIONS
DEVELOPMENT OF MORE SUITABLE LONG TERM CARE
FACILITIES AND HOME CARE SERVICES

inappropriateness of the existing mix of acute hospitals and crowded chronic care facilities for meeting needs of the disabled elderly and recommended development of more suitable institutional and home-based, long-term care services. A variety of innovations at the long-term care end of the health services spectrum ensued in the succeeding decades. A selection of these depicted in Figure 3 will be reviewed.

Foremost among the early initiatives was the forging of a formal linkage between the University of Rochester academic medical center and the large county infirmary (formerly poorhouse) to form a well-staffed chronic care institution, Monroe Community Hospital, in 1967. The intention was to provide the best of modern medicine to the hospital's large population of custodial care elderly patients and to provide multiple levels of long-term care appropriate to patient needs, from skilled nursing home to sheltered housing or placement at home with services (Williams, Izzo and Steel, 1975). Under vigorous medical directorship this hospital has achieved important successes toward this goal. This is reflected in an Evaluation-Placement project which among 332 consecutive patients referred for skilled nursing home level of care, was able to place the majority at lower levels of long-term care, many in their own homes. (Williams, Hill, Fairbank and Knox, 1973).

In 1975 building upon the demonstrated success of the Evaluation-Placement project, the Monroe County Long Term Care Program (ACCESS) was instituted as a Medicaid demonstration project to develop a community-based, efficient system for evaluating, and monitoring long-term placement for the disabled elderly. Acting as a brokerage service for patients classified as requiring long-term skilled level of care, in which case managers emphasize use of existing community services to facilitate maintaining patients in their homes, the ACCESS program has over a period of years successfully controlled rising costs for long-term care when compared with the experience of neighboring counties which lack such a program (Eggert, Bowlyow and Nichols, 1980).

Despite efforts of Monroe Community Hospital and ACCESS to meet the community's long-term care needs, the "backup" of elderly patients in acute hospital beds awaiting

FIGURE 3

HEALTH SERVICES FOR THE FRAIL ELDERLY
SELECTED INNOVATIONS - ROCHESTER

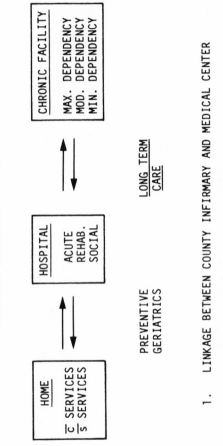

1. LINKAGE BETWEEN COUNTY INFIRMARY AND MEDICAL CENTER

2. MONROE COUNTY LONG TERM CARE PROGRAM (ACCESS)

3. GERIATRIC CONSULTATION ON ACUTE MEDICAL SERVICES

4. REIMBURSEMENT INCENTIVES FOR NURSING HOME PLACEMENT

nursing home placement became an increasing problem in the late 1970s (Rochester *Democrat and Chronicle,* 1982). This problem has been met by a number of further community-wide initiatives, emanating primarily from the ACCESS Program and from the Rochester Area Hospital Corporation (RAHC), an organization which coordinates planning and financing of acute hospital services in the area.

The first of these consisted of a one-year demonstration project funded by RAHC to establish geriatric consultation teams (physician, nurse, social worker) in each of the major acute hospitals in the county. The objective of the teams, modelled after the Edinburgh system described above, was to reduce prolonged hospital stay of high risk elderly "back-up" patients by providing consultation on rehabilitation and discharge planning early in the patient's hospital course. Over an initial six-month period, the census of elderly patients awaiting long-term care placement was reduced by 21% (Barker, Williams, Zimmer, VanBuren, Vincent and Pickrel, 1984). Formal consultative activities were discontinued with termination of project funding; nonetheless several participating hospitals are currently seeking means to establish more permanent geriatric rehabilitation services.

Both RAHC and ACCESS have developed special waiver programs with government third party payors with the object of expediting discharge of elderly patients with particularly heavy long-term care needs who are difficult to place in skilled nursing facilities. Under the RAHC initiative, which has yet to be implemented, hospitals would receive special capitation funds from third party payors with which to offer supplemental incentive payments to nursing homes (SNFs) to facilitate placement of such patients (Block, J. Personal Communication, 1983). Under the other financial initiative, known as ACCESS-Medicare, discharge of heavy care patients from hospital to SNF is expedited by waiving the initial Medicare approval process and guaranteeing Medicare skilled nursing level payment for at least the first two weeks in the SNF. Preliminary data indicate that proportionately more heavy care patients have been discharged to participating SNFs since the inception of this project (Eggert, G. Personal Communication, 1984).

SUMMARY AND DISCUSSION

This paper delineates a model of health services provided for elderly persons in industrialized societies and reviews the status and development of these services in two settings, representing two different societies. While essential components of primary care, acute hospital care and long-term institutional care are provided in both settings, it has been particularly instructive to observe the contrasting areas of emphasis in health service innovation with regard to the frail elderly. Rather than exhaustively reviewing all such developments, the paper is based upon a selection of exemplary undertakings from each setting. Furthermore, the paper focuses upon the conceptual and organizational aspects of these undertakings rather than a detailed critique of their measured impact on health or health services. (This information may be obtained from references cited.) What emerges is, on the one hand in Edinburgh, a consistent series of innovations emphasizing early intervention in health problems of the elderly in the community and avoidance of hospitalization; and on the other hand in Rochester, a consistent series of efforts to improve efficiency and appropriateness of placement of elderly patients in need of long-term care, with emphasis on home care in lieu of institutional care.

Explanations for the contrasting focus of health service innovation may be sought at national, regional and local levels in the respective societies.

Clearly the British National Health Service by providing comprehensive coverage for health services, has played a critical role in making possible the effective linking together of most components in the continuum of health services for the elderly. Furthermore, British health policy documents in recent years have repeatedly given particular attention to health needs of the elderly and emphasized strengthening care in the community (DHSS, 1976, 1978, 1981). In Scotland proper, a series of reports from the Royal College of Physicians, Edinburgh (1963, 1970, 1981) and the Scottish Home and Health Department (1980) have focused on ways to maintain elderly persons as healthy and independent as possible. The roles of general practitioners, community nurses and the home helps have been emphasized. Finally, given these facilitating factors, there has been strong and determined leadership in Edinburgh on the part of Professor James Williamson and colleagues in geriatric medicine to take the initiative to develop, test and teach the strategies of preventive geriatrics.

In the United States acute hospital and nursing home care, the two major components of health services for frail elderly persons, are largely financed by two distinctly separate programs, Medicare and Medicaid. Payment for long-term care elderly patients placed permanently in nursing homes or residing inappropriately in acute hospitals awaiting discharge to nursing homes has consumed increasing proportions of Medicare and particularly Medicaid dollars. Under these circumstances, cost containment of institutional services has been the principal concern of policy-makers, with comprehensiveness and coordination of services assuming secondary importance (Zawadski, 1983). Such concerns have been apparent for many years in the northeast region of the country which has proportionately more acute and long-term institutional beds than many other parts of the U.S. In recent years New York State health planners have focused upon the need for imaginative and efficient alternatives to the prevailing dominant and costly role of nursing homes and acute hospitals, albeit inappropriately, in providing for long-term care patients (New York State, 1979; Mossey, Cardillo and Goldman, 1983; Council on Health Care Financing, 1984). Innovative alternatives to institutional care have been stimulated by offering waivers to strict compliance with traditional requirements for third party reimbursement of long-term care.

The Rochester area with its long history of surveying and seeking community-wide solutions to the problem of inappropriate placement of elderly persons requiring long-term skilled nursing care has been a natural focus for undertaking such innovative projects (Zimmer, 1975; Finger Lakes Health Systems Agency, 1979). Rochester's impressive record in this regard has finally, as in Edinburgh, been critically dependent upon the active leadership of a core of talented health professionals committed to care of the elderly, in particular Dr. T. Franklin Williams, the first medical director of Monroe Community Hospital, who has played a significant role in all of the projects discussed earlier.

In the immediate future, the extensive experiences of Edinburgh and Rochester with innovations in preventive geriatrics and long-term care would appear to have much to offer to each other's societies. In the U.S., the current movement toward prospective systems for Medicare reimbursement of both hospitals and physicians, under Diagnostic Related Group and managed care programs, respectively, poses strong financial incentives to explore various community-oriented preventive geriatric strategies such as developed in Edinburgh. Furthermore, such strategies, which should prove far less costly and more appropriate than the traditional excessive reliance upon hospitals and nursing homes in the U.S., should be particularly attractive to Social Health Maintenance Organizations and the Veterans Administration in fulfilling their commitments to provide comprehensive health care for their elderly constituents. From the British perspective, the increasing proportion of very old persons is inevitably creating a greater burden of persons unable to be maintained in a preventive sense in the ocmmunity, hence calling for imaginative approaches to providing long-term care. Coordination between health, housing and social services at this end of the the care spectrum has been identified as a crucial issue to be addressed in the U.K. (Shegog, 1981). Herein, Rochester's extensive experience with multi-level institutional long-term care such as developed at Monroe Community Hospital and with community-wide brokerage of long-term care services such as that developed by the ACCESS program offers models which may well prove of value across the sea.

REFERENCES

Arcand, M., and Williamson, J. An evaluation of home visiting of patients by physicians in geriatric medicine. *British Medical Journal,* 1981, 3; 718–720.

Anderson, W. F. Preventive aspects of geriatric medicine. *Journal of the American Geriatrics Society,* 1974, 22; 385–392.

Barker, W. H. *Hospital-based geriatric services in Great Britain: Implications for the United States.* Report to World Health Organization, 1983. (Book manuscript in preparation.)

Barker, W. H. Survey of services for the elderly in general practices, Edinburgh. (Manuscript in preparation, 1984.)

Barker, W. H., Williams, T. F., Zimmer, J. G., VanBuren, C., Vincent, S. J., and Pickrel, S.G. Impact of geriatric consultation teams on 'back-up' of elderly patients in acute beds. (Submitted for publication, *Journal of American Geriatrics Society,* 1984.)

Brocklehurst, J. C. (ed.) *Geriatric care in advanced societies.* Lancaster: Medical and Technical Publishing Company, 1975.

Berg, R. L., Browning, F. E., Hill, J. G., and Wenkert, W. Assessing the health care needs of the aged. *Health Services Research,* 1970, 36–59.

Burley, L. E., Currie, C. T., Smith, R. G., and Williamson, J. Contribution from geriatric medicine within acute medical wards. *British Medical Journal,* 1979, 2; 90–92.

Council on Health Care Financing, New York State. Hospital alternate care patients in New York State. Staff paper. Albany, 1984.

Currie, C. T., Burley, L. E., Doull, C., Ravetz, C., Smith, R. G., and Williamson, J. A scheme of augmented home care for acutely and sub-acutely ill elderly patients: Report on pilot study. *Age and Ageing,* 1980, 9; 173–180.

Department of Health and Social Security. *Priorities for health and social services. A consultative document.* London: Her Majesty's Stationery Office, 1976.

Department of Health and Social Services. *A happier old age.* London: Her Majesty's Stationery Office, 1978.

Department of Health and Social Services. *Growing Older.* London: Her Majesty's Stationery Office, 1981.

Eggert, G. M., Bowlyow, J. E., and Nichols, C. W. Gaining control of the long term care system: First returns from the ACCESS experiment. *Gerontologist,* 1980, 20; 356–363.

Finger Lakes Health Systems Agency. Task force report on the hospital back-up of long term care patients. November, 1979.

Grundy, E. Demography and old age. *Journal of the American Geriatrics Society,* 1977, 31; 325–332.

Lowther, C. P., MacLeod, R. D., and Williamson J. Evaluation of early diagnostic services for the elderly. *British Medical Journal,* 1970, 2; 275–277.

Mossey W. L., Cardillo, A. D., and Goldman S. J. Providing an alternative to nursing home care: patient outcomes and costs in New York State's long term home health care program. Presentation at Annual Meeting of American Public Health Association, Dallas, 1983.

New York State Health Planning Commission. New York State Health Plan: *Long Term Care.* Albany, 1979, 123–149.

Rochester *Democrat and Chronicle.* "For old patients, nowhere to go." April 26, 1982.

Royal College of Physicians of Edinburgh. *The care of the elderly in Scotland.* Publication No. 22, 1963.

Royal College of Physicians of Edinburgh. *The care of the elderly in Scotland: A follow-up report.* Publication No. 37, 1970.

Royal College of Physicians of Edinburgh. *Appropriate care for the elderly: Some problems.* Publication No. 54, 1981.

Scottish Home and Health Department. *Scottish health authorities priorities for the eighties.* Her Majesty's Stationery Office, 1980.

Shanas, E., Townsend, P. Wedderburn, D., Friis, H., Milhoj, P., and Stehouwer, J. *Old people in three industrial societies.* New York: Atherton Press, 1968. Chapter 4.

Shegog, R. F. A. (ed). *The impending crisis of old age. A challenge to ingenuity.* Oxford: Oxford University Press, 1981.

Williams, T. F., Hill, J. G., Fairbank, M.D., and Knox, K. G. Appropriate placement of the chronically ill and aged. *Journal of the American Medical Association,* 1975, 226; 1332–1335.

Williams, T. F., Izzo, A. J., and Steel, R. K. Innovations in teaching about chronic illness and aging in a chronic disease hospital. In *Teaching of Chronic Illness and Aging,* Clarke, D. and Williams, T.F. (Eds) (NIH)75–876. Washington D.C.: U.S. Government Printing Office, 1975.

Williamson, J. Preventive aspects of geriatric medicine. *Modern Geriatrics*, October, 1970.

Williamson, J., Lowther, C. P., and Gray, S. The use of health visitors in preventive geriatrics. *Gerontologia Clinica*, 1966, 8; 362–69.

Williamson, J., Stokoe, I. H., Gray, S., Fisher, M., and Smith, A. Old people at home: Their unreported needs. *Lancet*, 1964, 1; 1117–1120.

Zawadski, R. T. The long term care demonstration projects: What they are and why they came into being. *Home Health Care Services Quarterly*, 1983, 4; 5–19.

Zimmer, J. G., and Berg, R. L. Data needs for regionalization. In *The regionalization of personal health services*. Saward, E. W. (ed.). New York: Prodist, 1975: 135–189.

Home Care of the Frail Elderly in the United Kingdom: Matching Resources to Needs

David Challis, BA, MSc
Bleddyn Davies, MA, DPhil

ABSTRACT. The paper reports the essential features and evaluation of a scheme to improve the effectiveness of home care for the frail elderly. Decisions about resource allocation were devolved to front line social work staff, giving them greater autonomy within clear expenditure parameters. More imaginative responses were noted in the management of a number of difficult problems and the results of the evaluation were generally positive. It appeared that the scheme was most cost-effective for the extremely mentally and physically frail living with others and also for the less frail, socially isolated, depressed elderly person.

An inevitable consequence of resource constraints, an ageing population and welfare objectives stressing the preference of many elderly people for care at home is the emergence of a long-term care population whose needs will have to be catered for in community settings, usually their own homes. Previously, it is likely that a considerable proportion of these individuals would have been cared for in residential homes or hospitals. This long-term care population is characterised by the variety of needs which must be met if care is to be adequate. Their needs are both extensive and intensive and vary because of the times at which help is required, the characteristics of

David Challis is Research Fellow, Personal Social Services Research Unit, University of Kent at Canterbury, Kent.

Bleddyn Davies is Professor of Social Policy and Director of the Personal Social Services Research Unit, University of Kent at Canterbury, Kent.

This research was made possible by Kent County Council, the Monument Trust and the Department of Health and Social Security.

their dependency which make different forms of assistance appropriate, the duration of required episodes of care, the amount of social support available and the mental health and personality characteristics which influence the ways in which help can be effective, to identify but a few aspects of variety. Consequently simply providing more care services is a necessary but insufficient condition, flexibility and appropriacy are also important. To respond effectively to the different aspects of need requires careful assessment and the construction of individual packages of care sensitive and unique to each elderly person. The services which are required to meet these needs are organisationally highly fragmented coming from a wide range of sources, both formal and informal, including the Social Services Department, the National Health Service, family, friends and neighbours. Indeed the picture of resource provision for the frail elderly is all too often that of a series of piecemeal interventions by a range of actors, none of whom have a clear responsibility for taking a broader overview of need beyond their particular remit. As a result services have been described as ". . . an uncoordinated set of discrete and relatively autonomous parts" and therefore ". . . the care which any individual old person receives is to a major extent fortuitous" (Plank 1977, p. 12). However, of all available resources, it is basic social care which is the largest single input for effective maintenance at home, as has been observed in intensive nursing care schemes (Currie et al., 1980; Gibbins et al., 1982).

The lack of any one person clearly responsible for cementing together these fragmented services into a coherent package is a significant factor militating against their capacity to prevent admission to institutional care. However, such an integrated system of care for an individual elderly person will not happen spontaneously, rather it has to be consciously created. Only where careful interweaving of the possible sources of help has been achieved is it possible for statutory help to function as a complement rather than a substitute for informal care (Moroney, 1976). The active building, support and maintenance of care networks to provide long-term care at home requires co-ordination, monitoring and adjustment of care by a specific individual or "key worker." In short this is effective case management of the kind that would be expected in child care services (Stevenson and Parsloe, 1978).

THE CHARACTERISTICS OF COMMUNITY CARE SCHEMES

The Community Care Schemes attempt to provide this improved case-management through a responsible social worker whose role includes making care at home more effective and achieving a more appropriate use of resources by increasing the range of choices open to an elderly person, delaying or obviating the need for unnecessary admission to residential care. The aim was that enhanced case management would lead to a closer focus of resources upon the most frail, an improved assessment of need, a more appropriate and individualized response to identified needs, continued monitoring and adjustment of resources to changes in circumstances by a "key" worker for an identified caseload of people.

The scheme introduced a number of devices to achieve these aims.

1. The social work staff appointed to the scheme were to have smaller caseloads than is usual in work with elderly people; their caseloads were to be similar to those of staff working with vulnerable children. This was to enable them to undertake more careful and extensive activity with elderly people, their relatives and others, careful ongoing assessment and monitoring, liaison with other services and investment of time in raising community resources such as neighbourly help or lodgings. Continuity of responsibility and specialisation in work with a particular client group should make possible an acquisition of knowledge which can produce an improved response over time.
2. The elderly people eligible for the scheme were to be those whose needs placed them at least at the margin of admission to residential homes.
3. In order to enable the workers to extend the range of possible responses to meet needs, they had control of a decentralised budget. This budget could be used upon services or developments necessary to support elderly people in the community and improve their quality of life. All the social services department's expenditure such as meals on wheels or home help was notionally

charged to the budget, as well as actual additional expenditures. In order to balance greater autonomy with accountability, expenditure upon individual cases was limited to two-thirds of the cost of a place in a residential home, expenditure beyond that limit requiring line-management sanction. Accordingly, knowledge of the unit costs of different services introduced an awareness of the relative costliness of different courses of action, which were previously seen as equally costly.

4. More experienced staff were to be recruited to work with elderly people. In many local authorities by contrast, relatively large and heterogeneous caseloads of elderly people tend to be managed by inexperienced or unqualified staff (Stevenson and Parsloe, 1978). Such large caseloads militate against continuity of contact and make less likely the kind of planned approach which can reduce the likelihood of crises and hurried admissions to institutional care.

5. The scheme area was wherever possible coterminous with the territory of other key actors such as the health service. As a result it was possible to build up a network of exchange relationships with people such as district nurses and consultant geriatricians in the deployment of domiciliary resources. This was to foster more effective cooperation and collaboration at the individual case level.

THE SCHEME AND CARE OF THE ELDERLY

In this section some of the scheme aspects which have influenced the delivery of care are considered. These factors include organisational location, assessment of need, the deployment of the budget upon community resources and responses to particular types of problem.

There has been some degree of variation in the position of the scheme within the Social Services Department in the different areas where it has developed. In the original scheme in East Kent a small team of social workers was established covering the same area as an area team. Further developments in Kent have located community care staff in area teams, whether organised on a generic or client group basis, for an elderly person's home and elsewhere the scheme is run as a separate small team. Nowhere yet has it been run from a hospital setting. Nevertheless, despite organisational differences there is a common philosophy and devices for the operation of schemes.

It was particularly noticeable that the greater flexibility of response afforded to social workers the provision of a decentralized budget provided an environment where *assessment of need* could be more effective. The approach has been "problem-orientated" rather than the assessment of elderly people in relation to their eligibility for a standard service. It therefore became possible to consider the identification of needs separately from the means of tackling them. Whilst the use of existing resources of the social services department has proved to be an important part of care for the majority of cases, these resources have been carefully interwoven with help from the local community. *The major new resource, developed with the budget,* has proved to be the use of local people as helpers, whether or not previously part of an elderly person's social network, to perform specified tasks for individuals usually for relatively small payments. The actual fee paid is agreed between the social worker and the individual helper and may vary according to the task to be done, the characteristics of the elderly person in question, the time at which the task is done and the circumstances of the helper. Payment is not for a given time but for the performance of the task. Whilst the provision of human caring resources is clearly an essential requirement for most of the elderly people, it was noticeable that this extra help has been on the whole recruited by the teams or was already part of an elderly person's social network and has not been provided through the private sector or voluntary agencies. Only in one rural area has an agreement been made to supply helpers through a voluntary agency, and even here this accounts for merely one helper in five.

Where helpers have been introduced to elderly people as part of a package of care the tasks to be undertaken have been made explicit in a "letter of agreement" which in effect clarifies the expectations of the social services department in providing a fee. The contract spells out the tasks to be undertaken in care and the objectives of care, providing some legitimacy and purpose at least in the early phase of client helper contact. This procedure makes the commitment regular and explicit, providing essential reliability for the elderly person and avoiding uncertainty for the helper has has been experienced in some volunteer schemes (Davies, 1977). Care has been taken to try and "match" elderly persons and helpers to attempt to ensure that both relational and instrumental needs are met. Helpers have ranged from those with previous caring experience, either professionally such as retired nurses or home helps, or informally within their own families, to those with room in their lives which they wished to fill with worthwhile activity, such as young housewives or the recently bereaved. The tasks which helpers have undertaken have ranged from immediately practical help with tasks of daily living to the social and therapeutic, such as accompanying a phobic old lady on walks of gradually increasing length, reactivating old interests and abilities or more simple companionship. One fifth of the specified tasks in the original scheme were purely social or therapeutic. These extra care inputs have been provided as part of an overall care plan, integrating the activities of several agencies, formal and informal carers.

As well as the use of the budget to introduce helpers to individual elderly people, it was catalytic in other activities. One of these has been the development of small day-care groups of four or five elderly people in a helpers home to undertake social and rehabilitative activities. This has proved particularly useful for people unsuited to more traditional forms of day care. Short-term care in helpers' homes has also been arranged following periods of illness or hospitalisation. In addition, the budget has been used to purchase aids or hardware not usually available. This has included the purchase of automatic electric kettles and oil-filled electric heaters for the use of demented elderly people, making it possible to reduce hazards such as a gas supply. Other purchases have included special vacuum flasks which can be used by those with arthritic hands and craft materials to encourage activities at home.

RESPONDING TO PARTICULAR PROBLEMS AND DIFFICULTIES

The position of the social worker as case-coordinator, able to make a flexible response to individual need by virtue of the possession of a budget has made possible a more appropriate response to a wide range of problems. This is described in more detail elsewhere (Challis, 1982; Challis and Davies, 1983) and it is only possible to make brief allusion here to some of the responses observed with difficulties which are frequently unresponsive to the usual range of services.

One factor which makes a considerable proportion of elderly people liable to enter residential care is *the risk of falling,* which by its very nature is unpredictable. Such unpredictability is a cause of concern to both an elderly person and their carers and may lead to an intolerable level of anxiety only resolved by admission to care. The uncertainty often results from the knowledge that visits are unpredictable, at infrequent intervals and the elderly person's expectation that if they fell they would have no knowledge of how long they would remain on the floor. The focus of intervention, apart from any alterations to the physical environment which might reduce the likelihood of falling, has to be tailored to the reduction of this threshold of fear. At times this could be accomplished by a regular, predictable pattern of visiting organised on a local basis, making the level of risk acceptable to the old person and their carers, in the knowledge that should they fall a visitor would be coming at a certain time. The risk of the damaging "long lie" (Hall, 1982) can thus be greatly reduced, and consequent pressures from relatives for an institutional solution may be reduced.

Elderly people suffering from *minor psychiatric disorders* such as depression, anxiety and alcohol-related problems are frequently recipients of insufficient resources in comparison with otherwise similarly needy people (Foster et al., 1976). It appeared that staff with great experience more frequently identified these problems and liaised more closely with health service personnel to obtain appropriate treatment. Consequently, with additional social support and stimulation accompanied by an attention to detail, a positive response was observed in a considerable proportion of those cases with depressed mood. A small but significant group, eight per cent of cases, suffered with problems of excessive alcohol intake, often in association with depression and social isolation. About half of these represented long-standing drink problems persisting into old age and the rest appeared to be of recent onset in response to social stress. With the former group, close support and supervision to maintain a level of acceptable or controlled drinking was reasonably successful, in part because sources of supply were known and could be controlled, and in addition attempts were made to mitigate the ill-effects of drink by ensuring the provision of an adequate diet. A similar strategy was adopted for the late onset individuals but the social workers also made greater efforts to relieve the precipitating stresses such as isolation and loneliness.

The care of the *dementing elderly* is perhaps the most demanding problem facing any home care scheme. The only evidence of predictors of success or failure in managing these patients at home is the Newcastle study which identified the importance of the degree and type of social support (Bergmann et al., 1978). Those living alone had the poorest prognosis, those with a spouse did better and those living with a younger family the best of all. The Community Care Scheme appeared to have some degree of success in terms of the establishment and maintenance of care and the reduction of risk to these individuals. The strategies adopted can be understood in terms of four factors. The first of these is the difficulty of gaining access or "entree" to the individual, and making help acceptable. This might require persistence, a response to particular behaviour problems, a willingness to initially provide help where perceived by the elderly person than where the need is greatest and an identification of those elements of retained ability as well as those areas of increasing deficits. The second and third factors represent different elements of risk. "Process risk" refers to the likelihood of increasing self-neglect, decline and reduction of coping skills, often a downward spiral. This was tackled by the organisation of care to provide supervision, food, medication and stimulation to arrest nutritional and social decline. "Event risk" refers to the loss of coping skills where normal sequential acts of daily living are not completed in their entirety, such as turning on gas taps and failing to light them, thereby causing a hazard to the elderly persons and their environment. This was tackled by modifications to the physical environment such as turning off the gas supply, identifying behaviour patterns and establishing routines with close supervision to reduce the risk of wandering. Whilst many individuals will exhibit a mixed picture of risk, the distinction has proved helpful as it serves to discriminate between different types and foci of intervention. The fourth element was "Patterning Care." This was the construction of a clear and regular pattern of care based initially upon the positive elements retained by the older person despite their mental disability. The pattern had to be meaningful within the old person's daily routine, or depend upon external cues such as light and dark, night and day. Where there was no such routine attempts were made to create one, for example, associating particular activities with retiring to bed, and perhaps tiring them at an appropriate time, so as to provide the person with a more predictable and apparently secure environment. In addition reality orientation approaches (Woods and Holden, 1981) were employed. Helpers were enjoined to convey information, such as the day of the week or the meal being eaten, in every interaction with the elderly person. With these cases a greater degree of direction was required of the social worker who had to take responsibility for providing a certain level and type of care and making it acceptable to the elderly person. Consequently the elderly person's decisions were less of a positive kind and more of a veto, as in the protective approach advocated by Wasser (1971). These responses were only possible due to the greater flexibility which was possible for community care scheme social workers.

Support for carers has proved to be another significant feature of Community Care Schemes. It may often be the case that existing services such as day hospital, day centres or home help are only partially effective, perhaps because an elderly person is too sick to attend or the carer does not desire help with domestic tasks. In certain cases what was required was help which fitted with the carer's particular interests, needs or problems such as regular relief on particular days or evenings, the stimulation of a visitor who could relieve both old person and carer or perhaps help to settle the old person at a specific time. At other times it was necessary to create boundaries for carers to reduce the effects of a gradually increasing burden and thereby to set limitations where possible to that commitment. The use of local helpers has provided the flexibility to respond in ways that range from simply sitting in with an elderly person to taking over the full care responsibility for several days each week. It did appear that the investment of appropriate help for carers at the right time enabled them to continue their caring role substantially longer than would otherwise have been the case.

Discharge from hospital and residential care has proved possible in a few cases, either earlier than would otherwise have been the case or from permanent care. This has been possible as the social workers have been able to plan these activities with sufficient control over resources to respond to the particular needs of individuals, and thereby gain the cooperation of hospital and residential care staff in planned rehabilitation and discharge.

SOME RESULTS FROM THE ORIGINAL COMMUNITY CARE SCHEME

Four of the Community Care Schemes are being evaluated, although results are only available for the first scheme in East Kent. The evaluation was undertaken using a quasi-experimental design and post selection matching, comparing similar cases from adjacent areas both of which were part of the same health and social care system (Davies and Challis, 1981). Interviews were undertaken with elderly people and their carers immediately prior to the scheme intervention and again one year later.

1. Destination of Cases Over One Year

Cases were matched by six factors likely to be predictors of survival in the Community. These were sex, age, living group (household composition), presence of confusion, physical disability and receptivity to help. As a result of this process 74 matched pairs were identified. The location of the 74 matched pairs after one year is shown in Table 1.

It can be seen that whereas 69% of the Community Care group remained in their own homes only 34% of the Control Group did so. This difference was largely to be explained by the different rates of admission to local authority care and death. Whilst these findings are broadly similar to those of an interim report (Challis and Davies, 1980) the death rate finding is new. However, since this effect was also present in the unmatched groups it was unlikely to be an artifact of the matching procedure. In the unmatched samples of 92 experimental and 116 controls, 67 per cent of Community Care cases remained at home compared with 45 per cent of the controls, and the death rates were 15 and 28 per cent respectively. No differences were evident between the groups in terms of functional status, incontinence, poor memory or other correlates of organic brain disease, and physical frailty was if anything greater for the Community Care Group. Two possible explanations for the differences in survival rate appeared to be the reduced 'relocation effect' (Yawney and Slover, 1973) since less of the Community Care cases entered institutional care and the influence of extended social support (Berkman and Syme, 1979; Parkes, 1980) for the Community Care group. A number of studies have indicated that the presence of a confidante can be a buffer mitigating the ill-effects of social stresses (Brown and Harris, 1978; Miller and Ingham, 1976). Therefore, at follow-up survivors in the community were asked whether they had anyone in whom they could confide. Whereas 58 per cent of the comparison group felt that they had no confidante only 15 per cent of the Community Care group felt this. Much of this difference was accounted for by the Community Care cases who would confide in their social worker or scheme helper. A similar survival pattern was also observed in favour of the Community Care Scheme over a subsequent three years (Challis and Davies, 1983).

2. *Quality of Life and Care of Survivors*

Tables 2 and 3 show the outcomes from interview data for quality of life and quality of care indicators. In each case the mean change, the difference between the first and second assessment for each variable is shown and the probability level of that difference, tested by analysis of variance.

It can be seen that there were significant improvements both in subjective well-being and quality of care for the recipients of Community Care compared with those elderly people in receipt of standard services. Only one of these indicators, "anxiety" failed to reach a satisfactory level of significance. This was because much of the evident anxiety was associated with risk to personal security amongst those who were socially isolated and at risk of falling. A considerable proportion of these in the control group were admitted to residential homes, which effectively reduced the anxiety associated with this risk. Hence there was no significant difference between the Community Care Scheme and standard provision for this factor. Other analyses demonstrated that there was a lower rate of decline in functional status amongst the Community Care Group, which could in part be attributed to close liaison between the scheme social workers and the Geriatric Day Hospital. No such close contact occurred for the control group cases.

There were also interesting results in the effects upon Principal Carers. Whereas the Community Care Scheme was significantly more effective in reducing subjective stress amongst carers, there was no significant difference between Community Care and the control group in relation to reduction in practical demands upon carers such as effects upon employment or social life. This can be seen from Table 4 where three of the subjective factors approached an acceptable significance level despite the small number, one in five, of cases with principal carers. The explanation for this appeared to be that, in the control group, elderly people with carers were particularly likely to enter institutional care. Entry to institutional care and effective support at home likewise reduce the difficulties in social life or employment. However a carer who has, through lack of any other option, had to place an elderly relative in institutional care may still experience guilt and distress. This was very evident in the interviews.

3. Costs and Cost Effectiveness

The costs of care were compared at 1977 price base, the year in which the scheme commenced. Costs are shown for the Social Services Department, the National Health Service

(NHS) and Society as a whole both as an annual cost and per month survived, since there was a difference in death rate between the two groups. The costs are shown in Table 5. These costs estimates are based upon revenue account expenditure by the two agencies and for social opportunity costs a 7 per cent discount rate was applied for capital elements.[1] Due to differences in accounting procedures, the agency costs for the social services department allow for capital costs but those for the Health Service do not. A capital allowance was therefore estimated as an assumption of upgrading of facilities for the NHS in the social cost computations. It was not possible to include family practitioner costs in the health service costing, but the difference in this between the two groups is likely to be small.

These average cost figures suggest a clear, if small, cost advantage to the Social Services Department from the Community Care Scheme. However, the NHS results suggest little difference in costs due to the two models of care, greater longevity tending to increase costs for the Community Care group. This average cost figure however conceals an important difference in its constituent parts. Whilst the Community Care Scheme tended to incur costs for the NHS in terms of acute admissions for short periods and Geriatric day care, much of the control group cost to the NHS lay in the use of long stay beds. Indeed, in the care of the very dependent, the Community Care Scheme appeared to be substituting for long-term hospital care, producing health care savings for this group.

Clearly the comparison of average costs and aggregate outcomes can only provide a very partial explanation of the results. The real question facing service providers, policy makers and planners is "For whom is this particular mode of care the most cost-effective response?" The answer to this question involves simultaneous examination of the relationship between costs, the characteristics and circumstances of individuals and the outcomes of care. This was tackled by the use of

---

[1]Social opportunity costs included Health and Social Care expenditures, the value of private housing and other resources consumed by the elderly person and financial costs borne by carers such as members of the family. The Capital costs of hospitals, residential homes and private housing were discounted over a 60 year period at a rate of 7 per cent.

multivariate statistical techniques to understand the influence upon variations in cost of individual client circumstances such as health, dependency and social support and two outcomes, subjective well-being and quality of care. The resultant cost equations clarified the effect of individual characteristics upon the process of care and could be used to predict the cost of achieving different levels of outcomes for different types of case.

It was observed that for costs to the Social Services Department that social support exerted a significant negative influence upon costs, that is to say the greater the degree of informal care the lower the cost of providing care and achieving improvements in quality of care. This was not the case for the comparison group. This was consistent with the development of complementarity between formal and informal care, described earlier, where an investment of support at the right time earlier and of the appropriate kind can reap considerable benefits through time. There was also a clearer costs by dependency gradient for the Community Care Scheme, indicative of a closer matching of resources to needs. In terms of costs to Society a negative effect upon costs of informal support was also observed for the Community Care Scheme.

The cost equations also served to tackle the cost-effectiveness question. These analyses suggested that there were two types of case for whom the Community Care Scheme was particularly cost-effective, both for the Social Services Department and for Society as a whole. The first was the extremely dependent elderly person with both mental and physical frailty who receives a considerable degree of informal support. This is consistent with the conclusions of Bergmann et al. (1978) who suggested that to focus home care resources on the demented elderly with informal support would be most productive, in view of the poor prognosis of those without informal support. The second group was the relatively isolated elderly person, with only a moderate degree of dependency, suffering from a non-psychotic psychiatric disorder, people whose difficulties may be particularly likely to remain undetected in usual circumstances (Kay et al., 1964; Foster et al., 1976).

Table 1 Location of Matched Cases after 1 Year

Outcome	Community Care		Control Group	
	N	%	N	%
Own Home	51	69	25	34
Local Authority Home	3	4	16	22
Private Care	6	8	4	5
Hospital Care	3	4	4	5
Died	10	14	24	33
Moved Away	1	1	1	1
	74	100	74	100

CONCLUSIONS

It would appear that the Community Care Scheme manages to provide an organisational context where what could be described as "good social work practice" with the elderly can develop. Creativity and flexibility may be less inhibited where devolution of control over resources to individual workers is possible within clear parameters of accountability set by expenditure guidelines. As a result the response is less the defensive posture of "guardian of scarce resources" and rather more that of "a discoverer and creator of resources" (Crosbie

Table 2   Quality of Life Factors

| Variable | Mean Change | | Significance |
	Community Care	Control Group	p
Morale	2.99	-1.00	< .001
Depressed Mood	-0.68	-0.17	< .05
Anxiety	-0.39	-0.2	NS
Loneliness	-1.46	0.36	< .001
Felt capacity to cope	5.03	0.66	< .001

et al., 1982). It would therefore appear that devolution of resources to the individual fieldworker is compatible with agency objectives where appropriate incentives are devised. Whilst the results in terms of costs and effectiveness appear satisfactory over a twelve month period there is always the possibility that over a longer period there will be a crossover point where care at home becomes more costly, or that over a longer time period different groups are more cost-effective. A follow-up of the original cohort of cases is now being undertaken to determine the costs and outcomes over a four year period.

The experience of the scheme in different parts of the United Kingdom has demonstrated that despite the arbitrary barriers that exist between health and social care, an improved service by one agency can provide benefits for both. However, given the complex inter-relationship between physical, psychiatric, social and emotional problems in the frail elderly there is room for an extension of this approach in terms of joint health and social services activity.

Table 3   Quality of Care Factors

| | Mean Change | | Significance |
Variable	Community Care	Control Group	p
Need for additional help night and morning	-0.58	0.13	< .05
Need for additional help with personal care	-9.47	-1.29	< .001
Need for additional help with domestic care	-6.68	-1.71	< .001
Increase in Social Contact	5.66	-0.77	< .001
Need for additional services	-2.44	0.69	< .001

Table 4   Outcomes for Principal Carers

VARIABLE		DESCRIPTIVE STATISTICS		
		Experiental	Control	Significance
1 Level of Subjective Burden	Mean	−1.12	−.33	.03
2 Extent of Strain	Mean	−1.24	−.5	.09
3 Mental Health Difficulties	Mean	−.82	−.25	.09
4 Difficulties in social life	Mean	−.71	−.67	NS
5 Difficulties in household routine	Mean	−.76	−.42	NS
6 Difficulties in Employment	Mean	−.18	−.01	NS
7 Financial Difficulties	Mean	−.12	−.25	NS
8 Difficulties with children	Mean	.06	−.17	NS
9 Physical Health Difficulties	Mean	−.41	−.33	NS

Table 5 Costs of Matched Pairs of cases

	Annual Cost £		Cost Per Month £ [1]	
	Comm. Care	Control	Comm. Care	Control
Social Services Department	638.95	701.74	51.54	58.56
National Health Service	778.00	707.81	68.98	74.92
Society as a Whole[2]	2850.02	2686.13	237.77	265.15

Footnotes:

1. Cost per month refers to per month survived. It therefore takes account of the shorter survival period of the control group.

2. Social opportunity costs included Health and Social Care expenditures, the value of private housing and other resources consumed by the elderly person and financial costs borne by carers such as members of the family due to factors like employment foregone. The Capital costs of hospitals, residential homes and private housing were discounted over a 60 year period at a rate of 7 per cent.

BIBLIOGRAPHY

Bergmann, K., Foster, E.M., Justice, A.W. and Matthews, V. "Management of the demented elderly patient in the community," *British Journal of Psychiatry,* 132, 441–9, 1978.

Berkmann, L.F. and Syme, S.L. "Social Networks, Host Resistance and Mortality: A nine year follow up of Alameda County Residents." *American Journal of Epidemiology,* 109, 186–204, 1979.

Brown, G.W. and Harris, T. "Social Origins of Depression." Tavistock, London, 1978.

Challis, D. and Davies, B. "A new approach to Community Care for the elderly." *British Journal of Social Work,* 10, 1–18, 1980.

Challis, D. "Towards more creative social work with the elderly." Stoke: University of Keele/Beth Johnson Foundation, 1982.

Challis, D. and Davies, B. "Matching Resources to Needs." Canterbury: PSSRU University of Kent, 1983.

Crosbie, D. "A role for anyone? A description of Social Work Activity with the elderly in two Area Offices." *British Journal of Social Work.* 13: 123–148, 1982.

Currie, C.T., Burley, L.E., Doull, C., Ravetz, C., Smith, R.G. and Williamson, J. "A scheme of augmented home care for acutely and sub-acutely ill elderly patients: Report on a pilot study." *Age and Ageing,* 9, 173–80, 1980.

Davies, B. and Challis, D. "A production-relations evaluation of the meeting of needs in the Community Care Projects" in Goldberg, E.M. and Connelly, N. (eds.), "Evaluative Research in Social Care." London: Heinemann, 1981.

Davies, M. "Support systems in social work." London: Routledge, 1977.

Foster, E.M., Kay, D.W.K. and Bergmann, K. "The characteristics of old people receiving and needing domiciliary services: The relevance of diagnosis." *Age and Ageing,* 5, 245–255, 1976.

Gibbins, F.J., Lee, M., Davison, P.R., O'Sullivan, P., Hutchinson, M., Murphy, D.R. and Ugwin, C.N. (1982): "Augmented Home Nursing as an alternative to hospital care for chronic elderly invalids." *British Medical Journal,* 330–333, 1982.

Hall, M.R.P. "Risk and Health Care." In Brearley, C.P. (ed.) "Risk and Ageing," London: Routledge, 1982.

Kay, D.W.K., Beamish, P. and Roth, M. "Old Age Mental Disorders in Newcastle Upon Tyne Part I: A study of prevalence." *British Journal of Psychiatry,* 110, 146–58, 1964.

Miller, P. and Ingham, J.G. "Friends, confidants and symptoms." *Social Psychiatry,* 11, 51–8, 1976.

Moroney, R. "The family and the state," London: Longmans, 1976.

Parkes, C.M., Benjamin, B. and Fitzgerald, R.C. "Broken hearts: A statistical study of increased mortality with widowers." *British Medical Journal,* 1: 740–743, 1969.

Plank, D. "Caring for the Elderly." London, *Greater London Council Research Memorandum,* 512, 1977.

Stevenson, O. and Parsloe, P. "Social Services Teams: The practitioners view," Her Majesty's Stationery Office.

Wasser, E. "Protective practice in serving the mentally impaired aged." *Social Casework,* 52, 510–22, 1971.

Woods, R.T. and Holden, U.P. "Reality Orientation." In B. Isaacs (ed), "Recent advances in Geriatric Medicine: 2." Edinburgh: Churchill-Livingstone, 1981.

Yawney, B. and Slover, D.L. "Relocation of the Elderly." *Social Work,* 18 May, 86–93, 1973.

Community Care of the Elderly in Britain: Value for Money?

Duncan Boldy, BSc(Hons), MSc, PhD
Reginald Canvin, BSc(Eng), MSc

ABSTRACT. An increased emphasis on community care for the elderly has been apparent in Britain for some time. However, if *appropriate levels of care* are provided at home and like patients are compared with like, residential care can be cheaper than community care. Nevertheless, if society places a value on maintaining the elderly in the community, rather than caring for them in institutions, then community care may well be value for money in this wider sense. However, we must not lose sight of the fact that value for money, and not just cheaper alternatives, is what we should always strive to attain.

INTRODUCTION

In most industrialised countries, the proportion of the population aged over 65 is greater than 10%. In England it is about 15%, having risen from about 10% since the time the National Health Service was introduced in 1948.

Because of their frailty, the elderly are major users of the caring services. As long ago as 1969 it was shown (Butterley, 1971), that the elderly, who then represented 13% of the population of England, accounted for 31% of health and social services expenditure. It therefore behooves us, from economic considerations alone, to examine whether we, or rather the elderly, are getting value for the nation's money, for the care provided for them.

Duncan Boldy is Senior Lecturer, Centre for Advanced Studies in Health Sciences, Western Australian Institute of Technology, and Reginald Canvin is Private Consultant, United Kingdom.

109

THE ELDERLY: WHAT ARE THEY LIKE?

The elderly are a very heterogeneous group. We probably all know frail old ladies of 65 and compare them (sympathetically or possibly even unfavourably) with active 75 year old gentlemen still tending their gardens. Not only are the elderly's needs different on the average from society's as a whole, but there are considerable differences between subgroups among them (Marshall, 1973). A chronological age of 65 years may be a necessary requirement for life membership of this club, but thereafter, age is not a helpful guide to the needs of its individual members. We must seek other criteria. We need to classify the elderly in such a way that each subgroup is defined unambiguously and in sufficient detail to enable professional case workers (e.g., consultants, senior nurses, senior social workers, etc.) to be able, from such a description, to prescribe appropriate forms of care for typical members in each sub-group.

Many classifications of the elderly have been developed over the years to help decide what services are required (e.g., Harris, 1971; Townsend, 1973; Wright, 1974; Burton and Dellinger, 1980) most of which include an assessment of the abilities to carry out specific tasks. One such classification used in Devon, England, and with modifications in other parts of England, is illustrated in Figure 1. By combining different levels of these characteristics and omitting some combinations which are unlikely to occur, or have similar care requirements, 32 operational categories have been defined and used.

THE CARE SPECTRUM

There are basically three broad types of long-term care provided for the elderly in Britain: long stay hospital care, residential home care and care at home by domiciliary services (principally home nurse, home help, meals on wheels) possibly supplemented by day hospital or day centre visits and/or warden support (sheltered housing). In the case of sheltered housing, a resident (or less often non-resident) warden acts as a "good neighbour", giving support in emer-

FIGURE 1

CLASSIFICATION OF THE ELDERLY USED FOR PLANNING PURPOSES IN DEVON

Characteristic	Brief Description
Physical disability	Four levels of ability to care for self and home
Incontinence	Four levels
Mental State	Three levels, depending on dementia and the presence or absence of behaviour disorder
Social Circumstances	Two levels, depending on the presence or absence of support from family and friends

gencies and arranging for services and aid to be provided as necessary. Table 1 shows how the elderly were distributed amongst these types of care in Devon in 1979 and indicates that there were more severely physically disabled people being cared for at home than in hospital. The purpose of this table is not comment on the provision in Devon but rather to give a flavour of the types of provision and the clients cared for.

Since the 1960s (Townsend, 1964), many research studies have shown that there is often inappropriate care provided for the elderly. As an example, studies carried out in Exeter, England (Canvin, Boldy and Taylor, 1972) showed that, of 170 long stay geriatric or psychiatric hospital patients, 23 (14%) could more appropriately have been cared for in a residential home, while of 420 residential home clients, 38 (9%) could have been more approporiately cared in a long stay hospital and 14 (3%) in sheltered housing. A more recent English survey (Cornwall and Isles of Scilly A.H.A., 1981) showed that of 1050 long stay geriatric and psychogeriatric hospital patents, 80 (8%) were considered to be more appropriate for residential home or domiciliary care, while 28% of residential home clients were considered to be more appropriately cared for in hospital.

TABLE 1
LOCATION OF CARE OF THE ELDERLY IN DEVON, 1979, BY PHYSICAL DISABILITY

Level of physical disability (1)	Percentage of total cared for				
	Long Stay Hospital (2)	Residential Home (3)	Sheltered Housing ± domiciliary &/or day care	Domiciliary &/or day care	Total
Severe	2.8	0.5	0.1	4.8	8.2
Moderate	3.0	3.6	0.3	9.7	16.6
Mild/None	0.4	6.3	5.4	63.2	75.2
Total	6.1	10.4	5.7	77.7	100.0

(1) Defined in terms of household and personal care ability (severe ▬ chairfast/bedfast; moderate ▬ personal care difficulties; mild ▬ household care difficulties)

(2) Geriatric or psychiatric

(3) L.A., private or voluntary

REASONS FOR INAPPROPRIATE CARE

There are many reasons why inappropriate care occurs, including the following:

a. a patient's, especially a long-term patient's, "needs" may change with time, but there is a conscious decision not to cause stress by moving the patient to a more appropriate form of care;

b. the provision of resources may not have followed the change in the number of elderly people and their changing "needs";

c. the most appropriate resource may not have been available at the time it was required.

A PLANNING FRAMEWORK

This imbalance of resources [(b) above] and/or "misallocation" [(c) above] stems in part from the fact that long stay hospitals, day hospitals and home nurses are provided by the health authority: residential homes, home helps, the meals service and day centres are provided by the Social Services Department of the local authority; while sheltered housing is generally provided by the Housing Department of a lower tier of local authority. Each agency has its own set of pressures, constraints and objectives and rarely is there an appropriate *framework* within which *joint* planning for the elderly can take place. In our view, it is not sufficient just to bring personnel from each agency together around a table and expect that a coordinated policy and plan will emerge from the ensuing discussions. They need appropriate *tools* to help them with their planning task.

One approach, called "Balance of Care" (Canvin et al. 1978; Boldy et al. 1981) uses a classification similar to that described above and requires professional advisers (health, social services and housing) to agree on possible alternative forms of care for typical patients in each category in the classification. Surveys indicate the existing care provided for patients in each category. The approach provides a means of calculating desirable changes in the provision of resources, given financial and other constraints and assumptions concerning the numbers of patients to be treated at some future time, say in five years.

In this way, the joint planning team is provided with a framework for their planning: a classification structure; the numbers of patients of each type receiving care; appropriate alternative forms of care; a joint review of different options. In developing this approach in Devon (and later in Cornwall) we placed particular emphasis on the opportunities which joint financing arrangements provided for shifting the balance of care towards the community. This has emphasised the desirability of increasing domiciliary and day care services—in line with DHSS recommendations (Department of Health and Social Security, 1981).

GAPS IN THE CARE SPECTRUM

Armed with this more analytical aproach to planning, it becomes easier to highlight gaps in the provision of resources; not only a shortage of existing resources, but possibly a need for somewhat different resources.

Various studies (e.g., Heumann and Boldy, 1982; Butler et al. 1979) have demonstrated the increasing ageing over time of many sheltered housing tenants. This trend, although not striking as yet, is showing signs of accelerating. It is due to the ageing of schemes, coupled with the (usually) conscious decision not to transfer tenants to residential homes or long stay hospital as they become frailer. A similar trend is also evident as regards the residents of residential homes (Department of Health and Social Security, 1982), in this case probably due in part to the demand for both residential home and long stay hospital beds exceeding the supply.

Figure 2 illustrates in simple terms our understanding of the existing situation, what we perceive as current broad trends and a possible alternative scenario; this we will now discuss.

One apparent gap in the present spectrum of care is seen as the need for the extra care provided by "very sheltered" housing schemes, with 24 hour staff surveillance by up to as many as four wardens and facilities for up to three meals a day for tenants; small nursing wings are even advocated by some authorities (Smith, 1980). The danger in this development is that all, or the majority, of sheltered housing schemes may become very sheltered, so that in filling the perceived gap between residential care and conventional sheltered housing, an even wider gap between very sheltered housing and the general elderly community may be opened up (see Figure 2).

One of us has demonstrated elsewhere (Heumann and Boldy, 1982), that sheltered housing in its original "good neighbour" form, can adequately care for a balanced mix of fit and frail tenants. The problem is that this balance is proving more and more difficult to sustain as schemes age and not enough new schemes are introduced. It is therefore almost inevitable that some schemes will be transformed into very sheltered schemes simply in order to care for existing tenants if they are not to be transferred to a residential home or hospital.

Turning now to the perceived gap between long stay hospital and residential home care, our survey carried out in Exeter (Canvin, Boldy and Taylor, 1972), showed that of 98 long stay geriatric hospital patients, 71 were considered by the geriatrician as more suitable for care in a residential home provided with some nursing care—i.e., a form of nursing

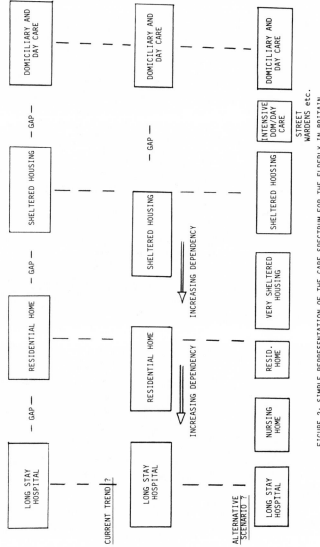

FIGURE 2: SIMPLE REPRESENTATION OF THE CARE SPECTRUM FOR THE ELDERLY IN BRITAIN

115

home. Such "bed-blocking" in long stay hospital has been recognised (e.g., Royal Commission on the NHS, 1979) and experimentation in the provision of NHS nursing homes, mainly staffed and run by nurses, has been recommended. Since, as we shall see, care in a long stay geriatric hospital costs roughly five times the care in a residential home—without nursing—there appears to be ample scope for providing a more cost-effective form of care for some elderly patients in the gap between hospital and residential home.

Finally, what of the gap between sheltered housing and domiciliary and/or day care? Increasingly, attention is being paid to alternative methods of "sheltering at home", using street wardens, alarm systems, intensive domiciliary care etc. (see e.g., Department of Health and Social Security, 1978). These have the objective of maintaining elderly clients in their own homes amid their familiar surroundings for as long as possible. Such schemes may cost more to run than sheltered housing schemes and possibly even more than very sheltered housing schemes because individual clients are dispersed. On the other hand, they maximise the possibility of family and voluntary help, thus reducing costs to the state. However, even if additional costs are involved, most people will consider them well worthwhile.

One view of any graded system of forms of care described above is that it should operate on a kind of conveyor belt system. That is, an elderly client would be transferred from one form of care to another as he or she becomes progressively more dependent. We do not share that view. Instead, the aim should be to enable the elderly person to remain in familiar surroundings as long as possible—maybe until they die there, in comfort and dignity. *If* a move is essential, then they should enter that form of care most suitable and acceptable to them at that time, where they might normally expect to end their days—again in comfort and dignity. "An institution which sets out to become a good place to die in, is likely to be a better place to live in . . . " (Miller and Gwynne, 1978).

The DHSS does not explicitly endorse this view but does nevertheless advocate an extended range of services for the elderly (and the mentally ill) as the following illustrates:

Care of elderly and mentally ill people requires a range of services from specialist hospital care through residential and day care, to support in the home. Smaller NHS units, nearer to home and family, would be more appropriate than hospital for many people, while others at present in residential homes would benefit from the provision of more very sheltered housing. Those local authority residential units which are too large to be ideal residential homes could be purchased by health authorities for use as NHS units and the funds transferred to the local authority in this way could be used to develop alternative provision. (Department of Health and Social Security, 1981, para. 7.3)

THE COST SPECTRUM

It was noted earlier that it is not at all straightforward to compare the costs of different types of care. The method adopted here is to compare the crude average annual running cost to the authority providing the service. This presents a problem, in that hospital running costs do not include capital, but local authority running costs of residential homes, for example, do and this must be borne in mind. (Also to be noted is that the cost of capital is not included in the running costs of sheltered housing.) However, hospital costs are so much greater than non-hospital costs, that whether or not capital is included in the hospital cost, is somewhat academic when making such comparisons.

In using the average cost method, we have made the simplifying assumption that the cost of caring for a very dependent person in hospital (or residential home) is the same as for a mildly dependent person. This assumption is not made in the case of domiciliary and day care however, because using the Balance of Care approach previously outlined, we have defined the desirable amount of each resource to be provided, and measured the amount that is actually given to clients of each category. We can thus indicate a range of domiciliary and day care costs covering the range of dependency assuming desirable levels of provision and another range related to current provision. (No attempt has been made to attach a cost to any family or friends contributions to community care of an elderly person; such contributions are often considerable.)

Figure 3 shows a comparison of these revenue costs of alternative methods of caring for the elderly, derived from the Balance of Care work in Devon, showing the cost of desirable and actual levels of provision. One clearly discernable feature is the big difference in costs between long stay hospital and residential care—even residential care plus nursing, as discussed earlier. This latter form of care must surely be worthy of more experiment as it appears to give so much more value for money than long stay hospitals for certain types of patient. (At the time of writing, a number of experimental projects are currently taking place in different locations).

Another outstanding feature is the very wide range of costs of geriatric day hospital plus domiciliary care. The high cost is associated with severely disabled patients who, if they are not in hospital, require a great deal of support (so much so that a local social worker suggested facetiously that the patient would probably die of hypothermia with the front door being constantly opened to let the carers in or out!). In addition, the cost of (ambulance) transport is a major component of the cost of day hospital care.

Thus, the overall picture illustrates that, if like patients are compared with like and *appropriate care is given at home,* residential care can be cheaper than domiciliary care. A Greater London Council study came to a similar conclusion, viz "when a comparison is made between persons of similar ability to care for themselves and receiving similar levels of care, the so-called cost advantages of domiciliary care and sheltered housing over local authority homes is reduced and perhaps completely disappears" (Plank, 1977). This is, of course, due in part to the fact that itinerant staff spend much of their time travelling and setting up their own "clinic" for each visit. Therefore each visit is expensive. Furthermore, a visit must be made—just in case—whereas a quick observation in a residential home or hospital may be all that is required.

Nevertheless, the Department of Health and Social Security probably reflects the general public's feeling in recommending an increased emphasis on domiciliary care, probably provided in purpose-built (sheltered) houses. Most elderly

FIGURE 3: REVENUE COSTS OF LONG TERM CARE OF THE ELDERLY IN BRITAIN (£1000) (1980 prices)

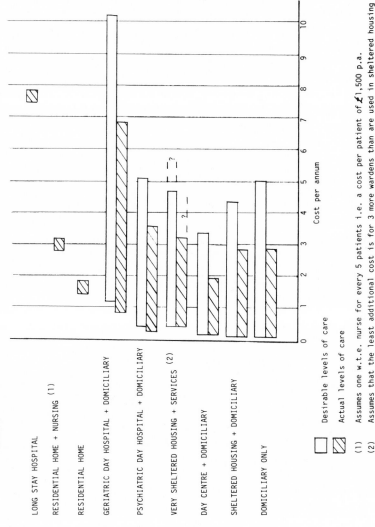

LONG STAY HOSPITAL

RESIDENTIAL HOME + NURSING (1)

RESIDENTIAL HOME

GERIATRIC DAY HOSPITAL + DOMICILIARY

PSYCHIATRIC DAY HOSPITAL + DOMICILIARY

VERY SHELTERED HOUSING + SERVICES (2)

DAY CENTRE + DOMICILIARY

SHELTERED HOUSING + DOMICILIARY

DOMICILIARY ONLY

Cost per annum

☐ Desirable levels of care

▨ Actual levels of care

(1) Assumes one w.t.e. nurse for every 5 patients i.e. a cost per patient of £1,500 p.a.
(2) Assumes that the least additional cost is for 3 more wardens than are used in sheltered housing

119

people appear to prefer it that way; the Greater London Council study already referred to (Plank, 1977) compared the preferences and attitudes of the elderly in sheltered housing, local authority residential homes and private households and found that those in sheltered housing were the most satisfied group. As we have seen above, this may be as expensive as, if not more so, than residential care, all else being equal; but if society places a value on maintaining the elderly in or near to their own home rather than caring for them in institutions, then that is the value we are getting for our money. It is value for money that we must be constantly seeking, not just cheaper alternatives.

REFERENCES

Boldy, D., Canvin, R., Russell, J. and Royston, G. Planning the Balance of Care, in Boldy, D. P. (Ed.), *Operational Research Applied to Health Services,* Croom Helm, London, pp. 84–108, 1981.

Burton, R.M. and Dellinger, D.C. Planning the care of the elderly, in Boldy, D.P. (Ed.), *Operational Research Applied to Health Services,* Croom Helm, London, pp. 129–155, 1980.

Butler, A., Oldman, C. and Wright, R. *Sheltered Housing for the Elderly; A critical review,* University of Leeds, Department of Social Policy and Administration, 1979.

Butterly, J. E. *Estimate of the total cost of the elderly for Health and Welfare Services in England 1968/69.* Institute of Biometry and Community Medicine, University of Exeter, England, 1971.

Canvin, R.W., Boldy, D.P. and Taylor, P.C.R. *The alternative forms of health and welfare care of old people in the Exeter and Mid-Devon Clinical Area.* Institute of Biometry and Community Medicine, University of Exeter, England, 1972.

Canvin, R.W., Hanson, J., Lyons, J. and Russell, J. Balance of Care in Devon; Joint strategic planning of health and social services at A.H.A. and county level, *Health & Social Service Journal.* pp. C17–C20, 18 Aug. 1978.

Cornwall and Isles of Scilly A.H.A. *Second report of the Care Planning Group for services for the elderly,* Internal Report, 1981.

Department of Health and Social Security. *Care in the Community,* H.M.S.O., London, 1981.

Department of Health and Social Security. *Statistics of Residential Accommodation of the Elderly and Younger Physically Handicapped at 31 March, 1981, England,* 1982.

Department of Health and Social Security. *A Happier Old Age,* H.M.S.O., London, 1978.

Harris, A. *Handicapped and Impaired in Great Britain,* H.M.S.O., London, 1971.

Heumann, L. and Boldy, D. *Housing for the Elderly—Planning and Policy Formulation in Western Europe and North America,* Croom Helm, 1982.

Marshall, T.H. The philosophy and history of need, in Canvin R.W. and Pearson N.G. (Eds.), *Needs of the elderly for health and welfare services,* University of Exeter, pp. 1–9, 1973.

Miller, E.J. and Gwynne, G.U. *A life apart.* Tavistock Publications, London, 1978.

Plank, D. *Caring for the Elderly: A report of a study of various means of caring for dependent elderly people in eight London boroughs.* Greater London Council, Research Memorandum, 1977.

Royal Commission on the N.H.S. *Report (The Merrison Committee).* Cmnd 7615, H.M.S.O., London, pp. 135–6, 1979.

Smith, P. *Ought there to be a future for very sheltered housing,* Centre on Environment for the Handicapped, London, 1980.

Townsend, P. The needs of the elderly and the planning of hospitals, in Canvin, R.W. and Pearson, N.G. (Eds.), *Needs of the elderly for health and welfare services,* Exeter University, pp. 47–70, 1973.

Townsend, P. *The Last Refuge,* Bell, London, 1964.

Wright, K.G. Alternative measures of the output of social programmes: the elderly, in Culyer, A.J. (Ed.), *Economic Policies and Social Goals,* St. Martin's Press, New York, pp. 239–272, 1974.

Health Insurance and Long-Term Care in Canada

William A. Mennie, MA

Health insurance and health care for long-term illness and disability in Canada are primarily the constitutional responsibility of the ten individual provinces. The organization and delivery of these programs is carried out mainly at the provincial and local levels, with the exception of certain federal services for special groups such as Indians and members of the Armed Forces. However, the federal spending power, which includes the right to make payments to the provinces, has played an important role in the development of provincial programs. Participating provinces remain responsible for program implementation and administration, but in order to receive federal financial contributions, each must meet certain national program conditions.

Long-term health care, which predominantly affects the elderly population, comprises a wide range of institutional and community services. At one end of the spectrum are the highly specialized services rendered by physicians in active treatment hospitals, and at the other end are the home help services that substitute directly for the traditional home responsibilities of families. Across this range, accessibility to the various components of these services in Canada has been governed by the shifting balance between the social security principles of *universality* and *selectivity*.

The principle of universality, of course, lies at the base of

William A. Mennie is Director, Health Economics and Data Analysis, Health Services and Promotion Branch, Health and Welfare Canada, Jeanne Mance Building, Tunney Past, Ottawa, Ontario, Canada K1A 1B4. This paper was presented at the conference session, "Health Insurance and Aging Populations: International Perspectives," at the 110th Annual meeting of the American Public Health Association, Montreal, Canada, November 14–18, 1982.

123

Canada's health insurance program. It is a fundamental program condition for federal financial contributions to provinces for health insurance that all residents of a participating province should be eligible for coverage of a national package of prepaid health care benefits. These include necessary inpatient public ward care in acute and chronic treatment hospitals under the Hospital Insurance and Diagnostic Services Act enacted in 1957, and all medically required services rendered by physicians under the 1966 Medical Care Act. Beyond these jointly financed basic insured services (plus jointly financed optional items such as hospital outpatient services), individual provinces have used their own financial resources to develop additional insured services. Provinces also operate separate workers' compensation programs for work-connected disease and disability.

The alternative principle of selective coverage on the basis of income status, derives from the traditional welfare approach. The Canada Assistance Plan, enacted in 1966, provides for federal financial contributions to provinces in respect of the cost of social assistance to persons in need, including the cost of health and social services that are not part of provincial health insurance plans.

CLASSIFICATION OF LONG-TERM CARE

For purposes of the following discussion, long-term care will be divided into institutional care (including hospital care) and non-institutional care.

Institutional care comprises the type of health care normally rendered in hospitals to inpatients, the lesser degree of care provided in nursing homes, and the personal support services in residential institutions, boarding homes and halfway houses. To avoid the confusion arising from a wide variety of terminology in different provinces, we shall rely mainly on the framework for classification of patient care (five categories) developed in 1973 by the Working Party on Patient Care Classification to the Federal-Provincial Advisory Committee on Hospital Insurance and Diagnostic Services.

Long-term hospital care (Type 3) is provided to a patient with a chronic illness or functional disability whose condition is no longer acute but whose vital processes may still be un-stable. Such a person may have limited potential for rehabili-tation but usually requires a variety of special services, medi-cal management and skilled nursing. This category should be distinguished from *rehabilitation care* (*Type 4*) applicable to patients with stable medical conditions requiring convales-cence or specialized rehabilitation services.

Nursing home intermediate care (*Type 2*) is furnished to patients with relatively stable chronic conditions who need little diagnosis and treatment, but are dependent on continu-ing skilled nursing and counselling. Such care usually lasts months or years.

Residential and boarding home care (Types 1 and 0) pro-vide support to frail persons who need help with the activities of daily living such as washing, dressing or cooking. Such care usually lasts several years.

Long-term institutional care for mental disorders involves any necessary combination of Types 3, 2, and 1 care for per-sons affected by mental illness or mental retardation.

Non-institutional care includes hospital outpatient service for ambulatory patients, services rendered by professionals such as physicians, organized community health services, and particularly, home care for long-term disorders.

NATIONAL HOSPITAL INSURANCE PROGRAM

Prior to the development of the national hospital insurance program in Canada in the late 1950's, there was relatively little provision by general hospitals for patients requiring long-term care; the financing of long stays was a critical prob-lem, and shortages of acute care beds accentuated the difficul-ties; patients with severe chronic conditions were shunted off to nursing home type institutions. Provincial welfare authori-ties paid the costs of such sheltered accommodation for indi-gent persons.

The 1957 federal Hospital Insurance and Diagnostic Ser-vices Act allowed for the inclusion of both acute and chronic hospitals in the national program of universal coverage hospi-tal insurance, but explicitly excluded tuberculosis sanatoria, mental hospitals, and nursing homes, homes for the aged and infirmaries providing custodial care. The cost sharing formula allowed for payment to provinces by the federal government of 25 percent of the provincial per capita cost of insured services (less authorized charges), plus 25% of the national average per capita cost, multiplied by the covered population of the province.

The inclusion of long-term chronic hospital care (Type-3) stimulated considerable upgrading of various institutional facilities in the provinces to permit their acceptance as federally cost-shared hospitals rendering insured services. Between 1958 and 1972 the number of chronic-convalescent beds in Canada doubled from 15,000 to 30,000, while acute short-term beds went up by 25 percent in the same period. The attractiveness of long-term care under hospital insurance, of course, was that patients not only did not pay charges on an ability to pay basis as in nursing homes, but could also retain their old age security income (if over 65 years of age). User charges in participating hospitals under hospital insurance were virtually non-existent because any such charges to patients for insured services required prior approval by federal Governor-in-Council, and even if accepted were partially deducted from the federal financial contribution to provinces. Thus, the program provided a financial incentive structure acting on patients and physicians which encouraged retention of long-term care patients in hospital, and in some provinces probably allowed a certain amount of lower level Type 2 care to creep into the hospital insurance system.

THE CANADA ASSISTANCE PLAN

The Canada Assistance Plan was the successor to the federal Unemployment Assistance Program which began in 1957 about the same time as the Hospital Insurance Program. This Unemployment Assistance Program included (among other things) 50:50 cost sharing with provinces of the basic maintenance costs of persons in financial need in what were termed "homes for special care." These facilities included nursing homes (Type 2), as well as residential and boarding home care facilities (Types 1 and 0). When the Canada Assistance Plan replaced the Unemployment Assistance Program in

1966, federal cost sharing was extended from basic maintenance costs, to include the cost of health and social services rendered to needy persons in these institutions.

The infusion of federal cost sharing funds plus rising income maintenance transfers for old age security and old age assistance (later the guaranteed income supplement), produced a dramatic increase in the supply of beds in homes for special care, particularly of the Types 1 and 0 varieties (i.e., residential and boarding home care). It would appear that the transfer payments enabled major increases in provincial rates of payment for indigent persons thus improving quality of care and encouraging an increased movement of low income frail elderly persons into institutional care arrangements. The sparse statistical data available suggests that between 1962 and 1972, beds for elderly Types 1 and 0 care may have increased from 23 to 42 beds per 1000 elderly population.

Nursing home intermediate care beds (Type 2) increased also but a less rapid pace, partly because the Hospital Insurance Program was stimulating conversion to Type 3 care. Between 1962 and 1972, the ratio of nursing beds in homes for special care per 1000 population 65 years of age and over moved up by 50 percent from 13 to about 20 per 1000. But some of this was a consequence of the transfer to homes for special care during this period of large numbers of long-term mental patients. Also, some of the smaller and poorer provinces found it financially advantageous to define border-line health care institutions as homes for special care rather than hospitals. Such provinces found the direct 50:50 cost sharing by federal and provincial governments under the Canada Assistance Plan for needy residents in homes for special care (there were relatively few self-pay cases in the poor provinces), to be more financially attractive than the slightly more than 25 percent marginal federal share of a higher cost under the hospital insurance financial formula.

The inclusion of many long-term patients with mental disorders in homes for special care, was a direct result of the explicit exclusion of mental hospitals from the federal-provincial hospital insurance arrangements in 1957. Under the Canada Assistance Plan in 1966, the cost of "persons in need" in any "home for special care" that was not defined as a hospital, was accepted for cost-sharing purposes. In some provinces, long-term care portions of mental institutions were separated and recognized as homes for special care, while in other provinces long-term patients were transferred to small residential facilities in various parts of the province. As regards institutional care for the mentally retarded, a transfer of jurisdiction to welfare departments in most provinces made it possible to consider these facilities as homes for special care rather than mental institutions. While patients were expected to pay in accordance with financial means, in practice the vast bulk of the patient population fitted the requirements of financial needs testing involving full support from public funds under the Canada Assistance Plan.

INSURED NURSING HOME INTERMEDIATE CARE

The provinces that had moved fastest in developing long-term hospital facilities under the Hospital Insurance Program began to find that perverse financial incentives for inappropriate higher level care were increasing the demand for beds faster than the growth in bed supply. Accordingly, some of them responded with an extension of the insurance principle (accompanied by uniform per diem user charges) to lower level types of care. Thus, came into being the Alberta Nursing Home Plan in 1964, the Ontario Extended Care Program in 1972, the Manitoba Personal Care Home Program in 1973, and the British Columbia Long-Term Care Program in 1978. Common features were prepaid coverage for Type 2 nursing home intermediate care, a standard daily user charge relating to the room and board component of care, income-related exemptions or reductions to the user charge, and a structure of formal assessment procedures for entry of clients into the programs. Additionally, the province of Saskatchewan introduced subsidies for the care of paying residents, later followed in 1981 by full public financing with a standard user charge; while Quebec reorganized most of its institutions as publicly financed "reception centres" in 1975 with a standard user charge feature.

As they extended the insurance principle to Type 2 care, some provinces experienced considerable difficulty in drawing a line between nursing home intermediate care (Type 2) and residential type care (Type 1). In many instances, of course, residents entering institutions for Type 1 care may graduate to more intensive care needs after a certain time. Furthermore, there was frequently a need for finer distinctions in care needs as a basis for provincial staffing standards and rates of payment to institutions. Several provinces developed their own classification system and terminology to distinguish additional levels of care, and to enable coverage of persons with somewhat lighter care needs. In general, the six provinces with some form of insured nursing home intermediate care have been more or less forced to include a significant number of Type 1 residents having moderate personal and supervisory care needs, within the framework of prepaid services and the standard user charge.

CONVERGENCE OF LONG-TERM HOSPITAL AND NURSING HOME CARE

By the early 1970's federal-provincial cost sharing arrangements under both the Hospital Insurance Program and the Canada Assistance Plan were perceived increasingly as barriers to rational long-term care policies in the provinces. Nursing homes were specifically excluded from coverage in the federal Hospital Insurance and Diagnostic Services Act, while simultaneously implementation of nursing home intermediate care insurance disqualified a province from cost sharing under the Canada Assistance Plan for care of needy persons in these institutions. Although special agreements were eventually negotiated with certain provinces to compensate them for the loss of cost sharing under the Canada Assistance Plan, pressures in favour of greater provincial flexibility increased. The result, in 1977 was the Fiscal Arrangements and Established Programs Financing Act which divorced federal financial contributions for health programs from provincial program costs, and instituted block funding arrangements involving escalation of federal contributions in relation to GNP growth.

The new federal-provincial arrangements for hospital insurance and medical care, retained the essential program conditions of universal coverage, comprehensiveness of benefits, reasonable accessibility, portability and public administration, in return for uniform per capita federal financial contributions to provinces composed of a mix of cash and tax room transfers. At the same time, a new uniform per capita Extended Health Care Services cash contribution without program conditions, was established to replace Canada Assistance Plan cost sharing related to institutions providing nursing home intermediate care, adult residential care, ambulatory health services, and home health care services. The provinces were well pleased. Aggregate federal funding for the overall health care package had been increased (the total by 1981-82 was $7.6 billion), while provinces now had full flexibility to support the defined extended health care services either on an insurance basis or a social assistance basis.

One important consequence in the central and western provinces has been a process of convergence towards essentially similar prepayment arrangements for long-term hospital and nursing home care (Types 3 and 2), as well as some adult residential care (Type 1). This was because the practical sanctions in the federal legislation against hospital user charges were gone. Although the federal program condition of "reasonable access" to insured services without preclusion or impediment, financial or otherwise, remained in force, no longer were hospital user charges deducted in part from the federal financial contribution, and no longer did they require prior approval by Governor-in-Council. The result for long-term hospital care has been a new structure of standard per diem user charges, applicable mainly to the room and board component, and broadly equivalent in amount to the income of a single person receiving old age security and the full guaranteed income supplement. By 1982, virtually all Type 3 and Type 2 standard ward care (and some Type 1 care) in each of the six provinces was being financed from public funds, with a common daily user charge for standard ward accommodation ranging in mid 1982 from $8.00 a day in Alberta to $13.80 a day in Ontario. For patients lacking the ability to pay the user charge, notably the adult mentally ill and retarded under the age of 65, there are exemptions or reductions based on income status.

In the four Atlantic Provinces, on the other hand, the social assistance approach has remained largely intact. The unconditional federal Extended Health Services Grant (totalling $0.7 billion for all provinces in 1981–82) has not been sufficient to stimulate movement towards the insurance approach, which would also require costly expansion and upgrading of facilities. Thus, Type 2 and 1 care, and much of Type 3 care, has continued to be provided on an ability to pay basis, plus public financing as required on behalf of persons in need. It may be noted, also, that in all provinces, Type 1 residential care for children, (the mentally retarded being the most numerous) continues on a social assistance basis, because this group continues to be cost shared through the Canada Assistance Plan.

NON-INSTITUTIONAL CARE

Of course, it has long been recognized that services in the community offer a preferable alternative to institutional care for many persons affected by serious long-term illness and disability. The ultimate question, however, has been whether community services are cheaper as well as therapeutically more beneficial.

For ambulatory patients, the issue was never in doubt, and Canada's health insurance arrangements have reflected this fact. Within the scope of the national health insurance program are insured out-patient benefits provided through the general and special out-patient clinics and emergency departments of general hospitals under the Hospital Insurance and Diagnostic Services Act; and all medically necessary services rendered by physicians within or outside hospitals under the Medical Care Act. Jointly financed by federal and provincial governments, these insured services constitute a nation-wide basic benefit structure for ambulatory care. Moreover, using their own financial resources, various provinces have developed additional insured benefit programs of relevance to long-term care such as: prescription drug benefit programs, prosthetic and orthotic appliances and hearing aids, ambulance services, and paramedical services such as chiropractic, optometry, podiatry and out-of-hospital physiotherapy.

For the less ambulant long-term multi-problem patient, the question of treatment and support services delivered at home has been more problematical. Until recent years support in the home in most parts of Canada comprised a bewilderingly fragmented mixture of health and social services delivered by a great variety of local voluntary groups, welfare agencies, health departments and visiting nurse organizations. The focus was on low income clientele, the funding came from charitable contributions and provincial governments, and availability of services tended to vary widely in different geographic areas. The selective social assistance approach, with federal cost sharing under the Canada Assistance Plan, was palliative in nature, and seemed to have slight impact in restraining the rapid growth of institutional care prior to the mid-1970's.

The coordinated delivery of professional health care and other support services to the home was started experimentally in some local areas as an offshoot of the Hospital Insurance Program. Despite the absence of direct federal cost sharing, except for some demonstration project grants, a number of provinces initiated home care programs that tended to concentrate on short-term care for acute treatment patients. The more complex and costly long-term care patients were largely ignored (with some exceptions) until the coming of the new insured nursing home intermediate care programs in the central and western provinces, mainly in the 1970's.

Both the cost containment and quality of care objectives of the new programs motivated the accompanying development of new province-wide structures for formal assessment and appropriate placement of applicants for admission, which could not overlook the home care option. It became apparent that the financial incentives to institutional care acting on patients and their families could only be offset by free-of-charge insured services in the home, including not only professional health care but homemaker and other support services needed in particular cases. And thus began the comprehensive Manitoba and Quebec home care program in the mid-seventies, the British Columbia, Alberta and Saskatchewan programs in 1978, and the Ontario chronic home care program launched experimentally in 1975 with province-wide extensions announced for 1982. The federal government gave its "imprimatur" by including home care within the parameters of the Extended Health Care Services contribution, although no program conditions were attached.

The principle of universally covered prepaid home care has, therefore, been established for long-term care patients who are assessed as meeting the medical necessity requirements and other criteria, and who live in areas where the services are available in the six provinces. A full range of professional health services, plus drugs, dressings, equipment etc., and even including homemaking services, are free of charge in Quebec and Manitoba. The same applies in British Columbia and Ontario, except for some monthly hours of work limits on home making assistance in Ontario, and some limits on services to persons under 65 years of age in British Columbia. In Saskatchewan and Alberta there are user charges with arrangements for subsidization based on family income and amount of service received.

Again, as for institutional care, organized home care programs have remained relatively undeveloped in the Atlantic Provinces. Services have been set up in some urban areas, but public financing is limited mainly to traditional local health unit services in the home. The social assistance approach continues, in the absence of insurance coverage for long-term care in institutions.

CONCLUDING REMARKS

The progressive extension of the insurance principle of prepaid care to a broader range of services in various provinces of Canada has improved accessibility to services and the quality of care rendered to persons affected by long-term illness and disability.

Accompanying this extension has been the growth of organizational structures aiming at more appropriate placement and location of patients in accordance with socio-medical need. Such structures are essential for cost effective resource allocation at a time of rapidly increasing demand for long-term care, in an era of financial constraint. Cost containment efforts by provinces, however, are being further tightened by supply control measures such as definition of "allowable" number of beds, restriction of new construction, and cut backs in allocation of resources. Thus, paradoxically, the growth of benefit coverage may have slowed the growth of resource allocation to long-term care. For example, the available statistics suggest that the current ratio of about 80 institutional long term care beds per 1000 elderly persons have changed very little from the early 1970's, by contrast with rapid earlier increases in the 1960's when "social assistance" financing prevailed. But, a much higher proportion of these beds, apparently are occupied by "heavy care" Types 3 and 2 clientele, while "lighter care" persons are remaining in their own homes to a greater degree. Similarly, the coordinated home care machinery permits the allocation of limited resources in accordance with socio-medical need criteria.

Many problems remain such as the insufficiency of total resources allocation, the lack of full coverage in the Atlantic Provinces and some parts of other provinces, and the frictional difficulties of matching individual care needs with appropriate resources. However, a hopeful sign that long-term care patients are beginning to get a better deal are the expenditure trends. In fiscal year 1981–82, estimated provincial government spending on long-term institutional and home care (excluding hospital care) was $2.6 billion compared to about $1 billion six years earlier in 1975–76. Such spending on long term care has moved up from 8.6 percent of all provincial government health spending in 1975 to 11.3 percent in 1981.

An Evaluation of the Role,
Theory, and Practice
of the Occupation of Homemaker

Jane Auman, RN, MA
Robert Conry, PhD

ABSTRACT. Homemaker service is currently used throughout Canada as a way of extending health care and social service assistance to certain clients. While the utilization of homemaker service has been increasing dramatically in the last decade, there have been no studies that have attempted to look at the congruency or discrepancy between what the homemaker is trained to do and what·she actually does in practice within the home of the client. This study, conducted in the lower mainland of British Columbia in 1981 presents such an evaluative analysis of the homemaker.

INTRODUCTION

Homemaker service is currently utilized in North America and in some European countries as a way of extending health care and housekeeping assistance to certain clients. This study looks at the overall theory of homemaker services and training, and the discrepancies that appear to exist in certain areas of practice and training. The most notable areas of discrepancy were found to be in the health care service categories of the homemakers' assisting with medication administration, replacing Home Care nurses, and the monitoring of clients' states of health.

Ms. Auman is a doctoral candidate in the Department of Mathematics and Science Education, The University of British Columbia. Dr. Conry is an Associate Professor in the Department of Educational Psychology and Special Education, The University of British Columbia.

Background to Contemporary Homemaker Utilization

The homemaker agencies are a collection of various non-profit and profit associations that provide housekeeping and health care assistance to certain clients. These associations were originally created within the professional mode of social service assistance to those in need in the early nineteen hundreds. This form of assistance has been increasing rapidly in response to accelerating demands for assistance to the elderly, the chronically ill, and the dependent individuals within society. In many instances clients are offered a choice between homemaker assistance in their homes or the alternative of institutional care outside of the home. Such assistance has been viewed by many as a means of providing health care and social assistance to the client while minimizing delivery costs to the taxpayers (MacIntyre, 1977; Robinson, 1974; Canadian Council on Social Development, 1971).

Although utilization of homemaker services has been increasing across North America, especially within the last decade, there have been few studies that have attempted to analyze or assess this unique form of client assistance. The purpose of this study was to trace the development of homemaker services in British Columbia, to delineate the understandings that people have about the concept of the homemaker, and to find the discrepancies that exist between certain areas of homemaker training and homemaker practice. The study presented here involved an in-depth analysis of two hundred randomly selected homemaker client files from the largest homemaker agency in the Province of British Columbia. The actual curriculum that was taught to this agency's homemakers was compared with the categories of practice performed in the homes of these clients. A Provus (1971) "discrepancy model" was implemented to identify areas of congruency and discrepancy between training and practice. Interviews with homemaker supervisors were also conducted to illuminate the discrepancies which appeared between the theory, as manifested in the training program, and the actual practice of the homemaker in the home of the client.

METHODOLOGY

The research was conducted using the following methodologies: content analysis of homemaker client files, content analysis of homemaker supervisor interviews, a Provus (1971) discrepancy model analysis of homemaker curriculum and homemaker practices, and a documentary analysis of reports and newspaper articles related to homemaker services.

Sampling

For the purpose of comparison, two hundred client files each from 1976 and 1980 were randomly selected. The total number of client files contained within the agency researched were approximately two thousand. The years 1976 and 1980 were chosen so that the role and practice of the homemaker could be assessed prior to and following the introduction of Long Term Care Legislation in 1978 within the Province of British Columbia. Once the information had been retrieved, content analysis was then employed as a means of reducing the information to the form of smaller, mutually exclusive units. The broad categories were either biodemographic in nature, relating to client or client characteristics or were categories related to actual homemaker practice in the home in which services of a health care or housekeeping assistance were being performed. After classification these categories were then statistically compared.

The next step was to compare the practice categories obtained with the 1980 curriculum of the homemaker training program. The Provus Discrepancy Model (Provus, 1971) was employed for this purpose. The Provus Model is an evaluative framework for analyzing congruence and/or discrepancy between desired and existing practices such as curricular theory and professional practice. The Provus Model has five stages:

Stage I: Design of the Program;
Stage II: Program Instillation and Congruence Testing;
Stage III: Delineation of Interim Products;
Stage IV: Terminal Products;
Stage V: Cost Effectiveness of the Program.

In the final step focussed interviews were conducted with a representative sampling of twenty percent of the total homemaker supervisory staff. Supervisors in half hour interview sessions were asked to comment on the training of their homemaker staff and specifically to give their own views regarding discrepancy and/or congruency that exists between homemaker training and the actual homemaker practice within the client's home.

These methods described above were selected in order to provide a multidimensional view of the homemaker's role, theory, and practice within the specified period of time, and to generate "observations" compatible in form with the intents of the Provus Discrepancy Model.

RESULTS

Overview

In general, the findings of this study provide a composite picture of a specific group of homemakers and their clients in which there has been significant change within the last decade. The role and practice of the homemaker appears to have undergone systematic alterations. In several instances, the curricular theory underlying their training programs does not match current practices. However, the results include more indicators of congruency than discrepancy.

Biodemographic Changes

An analysis of the data reveals that the typical homemaker clients of 1980 were, on average, older than their 1976 counterparts. Also, clients of 1980 were found in smaller family units, had a significantly higher degree of psychiatric and medical problems. This client of 1980 also presented fewer requests for child care assistance than did the client of 1976.

Congruence and Discrepancy in Theory and Practice

Congruency between the theory of the homemaker training program's curriculum and the actual practice of the homemaker in the client's home were found to exist in eight of the

Table 1

Cross Tabulation of Sex and Year

	1976		1980		1980(LTC)[1]		1980(not LTC)	
	f	%	f	%	f	%	f	%
Male	11	(11.1)	19	(19.0)	8	(20.5)	11	(18.0)
Female	87	(87.9)	79	(79.0)	31	(79.5)	48	(78.7)
Couple	1	(1.0)	2	(2.0)	0	(0.0)	2	(3.3)
Total	99		100		39		61	

Significance Tests

1976 vs. 1980	= 2.847 (df = 2; P = 0.241).
1976 vs. 1980(not LTC)	= 2.729 (df = 2; P = 0.255).
1980(LTC) vs. 1980(not LTC)	= 1.358 (df = 2; P = 0.507).

[1]Long term care

Table 2

Cross Tabulation of Age and Year

years	1976 f	1976 %	1980 f	1980 %	1980(LTC) f	1980(LTC) %	1980(not LTC) f	1980(not LTC) %
10 - 19	0	(0.0)	1	(1.2)	0	(0.0)	1	(2.0)
20 - 29	23	(25.0)	8	(9.4)	0	(0.0)	8	(16.3)
30 - 39	19	(20.7)	6	(7.1)	0	(0.0)	6	(12.2)
40 - 49	3	(3.3)	4	(4.7)	0	(0.0)	4	(8.2)
50 - 59	8	(8.7)	7	(8.2)	3	(8.3)	4	(8.2)
60 - 69	9	(9.8)	20	(23.5)	10	(27.8)	10	(20.4)
70 - 79	17	(18.5)	16	(18.8)	6	(16.7)	10	(20.4)
80 - 89	9	(9.8)	22	(25.9)	17	(47.2)	5	(10.2)
90 - 99	4	(4.3)	1	(1.2)	0	(0.0)	1	(2.0)
Total	92		85		36		49	

Significance Tests

1976 vs. 1980	Kendall's Tau C =	0.281; (P = 0.001).
1976 vs. 1980(not LTC)	Kendall's Tau C =	0.077; (P = 0.414).
1980(LTC) vs. 1980(not LTC)	Kendall's Tau C =	-0.512; (P = 0.000).

Table 3

Cross Tabulation of Number in Family Unit and Year

no.	1976 f	%	1980 f	%	1980(LTC) f	%	1980(not LTC) f	%
1	41	(41.4)	46	(46.5)	26	(68.4)	20	(32.8)
2	15	(15.2)	29	(29.3)	11	(28.9)	18	(29.5)
3	22	(22.2)	10	(10.1)	1	(2.6)	9	(14.8)
4	7	(7.1)	8	(8.1)	0	(0.0)	8	(13.1)
5	6	(6.1)	2	(2.0)	0	(0.0)	2	(3.3)
6	7	(7.1)	1	(1.0)	0	(0.0)	1	(1.6)
7	1	(1.0)	3	(3.0)	0	(0.0)	3	(4.9)
Total	99		99		38		61	

Significance Tests

1976 vs. 1980   Kendall's Tau C = -0.135; (P = 0.087).
1976 vs. 1980(not LTC)   Kendall's Tau C = 0.026; (P = 0.777).
1980(LTC) vs. 1980(not LTC) Kendall's Tau C = 0.439; (P = 0.000).

Table 4

Cross Tabulation of Method of Referral and Year

Method of Referral

	1976		1980		1980(not LTC)	
	f	%	f	%	f	%
Long Term Care (LTC)	0	(0.0)	39	(43.3)	–	
Client/Relative of Client	39	(39.8)	3	(3.3)	3	(5.9)
Medical Staff	23	(23.5)	19	(21.1)	19	(37.3)
Social Service Agency	36	(36.7)	29	(32.2)	29	(56.9)
Total	98		90		51	

Significance Tests

1976 vs. 1980   = 70.78 (df = 3; P = 0.000).
1976 vs. 1980(not LTC) = 19.06 (df = 2; P = 0.000).

Table 5

Cross Tabulation of Combined Personal Care Practice and Year

Client received Personal Care	1976		1980		1980(LTC)		1980(not LTC)	
	f	%	f	%	f	%	f	%
No	87	(87.0)	58	(58.0)	17	(43.6)	41	(67.2)
Yes	13	(13.0)	42	(42.0)	22	(56.4)	20	(32.8)
Total	100		100		39		61	

Significance Tests

1976	vs.	1980 = 21.09 (df = 1; P = 0.000).
1976	vs.	1980(not LTC) = 9.103 (df = 1; P = 0.003).
1980(LTC)	vs.	1980(not LTC) = 5.450 (df = 1; P = 0.020).

Table 6

Cross Tabulation of Combined Child Care Practice and Year

Client received Child Care	1976 f	1976 %	1980 f	1980 %	1980(LTC) f	1980(LTC) %	1980(not LTC) f	1980(not LTC) %
No	55	(55.0)	81	(81.0)	39	(100.)	42	(68.9)
Yes	45	(45.0)	19	(19.0)	0	(0.0)	19	(31.1)
Total	100		100		39		61	

Significance Tests

1976   vs. 1980   = 15.53 (df = 1; P = 0.000).
1976   vs. 1980(not LTC)   = 3.036 (df = 1; P = 0.082).
1980(LTC)   vs. 1980(not LTC)   = 15.00 (df = 1; P = 0.000).

Table 7

Cross Tabulation of Combined Housekeeping Practice and Year

Client received Housekeeping	1976		1980		1980(LTC)		1980(not LTC)	
	f	%	f	%	f	%	f	%
No	7	(7.0)	3	(3.0)	3	(7.7)	0	(0.0)
Yes	93	(93.0)	97	(97.0)	36	(92.3)	61	(100.)
Total	100		100		39		61	

Significance Tests

1976	vs.	1980	= 1.684	(df = 1;	P = 0.194).
1976	vs.	1980(not LTC)	= 4.464	(df = 1;	P = 0.035).
1980(LTC)	vs.	1980(not LTC)	= 4.837	(df = 1;	P = 0.028).

Table 8

Cross Tabulation of Combined Psychiatric Problems and Year

Client indicated Psychiatric Problems	1976		1980		1980(LTC)		1980(not LTC)	
	f	%	f	%	f	%	f	%
No	92	(92.0)	80	(80.0)	36	(92.3)	44	(72.1)
Yes	8	(8.0)	20	(20.0)	3	(7.7)	17	(27.9)
Total	100		100		39		61	

Significance Tests

1976 vs. 1980	= 5.980	(df = 1; P = 0.015).
1976 vs. 1980(not LTC)	= 11.40	(df = 1; P = 0.001).
1980(LTC) vs. 1980(not LTC)	= 6.053	(df = 1; P = 0.014).

Table 9

Cross Tabulation of Combined Medical Problems and Year

Client indicated Medical Problems	1976		1980		1980(LTC)		1980(not LTC)	
	f	%	f	%	f	%	f	%
No	35	(35.0)	20	(20.0)	2	(5.1)	18	(29.5)
Yes	65	(65.0)	80	(80.0)	37	(94.9)	43	(70.5)
Total	100		100		39		61	

Significance Tests

1976   vs. 1980   = 5.643 (df = 1; P = 0.018).
1976   vs. 1980(not LTC) = 0.517 (df = 1; P = 0.472).
1980(LTC) vs. 1980(not LTC) = 8.838 (df = 1; P = 0.003).

147

Table 10

Cross Tabulation of Child Care Problems and Year

Client indicated Child Care Problems	1976 f	1976 %	1980 f	1980 %	1980(LTC) f	1980(LTC) %	1980(not LTC) f	1980(not LTC) %
No	72	(72.0)	94	(94.0)	39	(100.)	55	(90.2)
Yes	28	(28.0)	6	(6.0)	0	(0.0)	6	(9.8)
Total	100		100		39		61	

Significance Tests

1976   vs. 1980   = 17.15 (df = 1; P = 0.000).
1976   vs. 1980(not LTC)   = 7.504 (df = 1; P = 0.006).
1980(LTC) vs. 1980(not LTC)   = 4.081 (df = 1; P = 0.043).

eleven categories tabulated from the data. The categories of congruence were: Ambulate Client, Help Dress, Help Bathe, Care for Children, Clean, Do Laundry, Prepare Meals, and Shop for Groceries. Discrepancy between curricular theory and practice existed in the categories of: Monitor Client's State of Health, Assist with Medication, and Replace Home Care Nurse on a Temporary Basis.

Summary of the Statistical Data

The statistical analysis was constructed to reflect the following: biodemographic profiles of typical clients; the reasons they received homemaker service; and what kinds of homemaker assistance were provided to these clients.

The homemaker practice and client diagnosis categories were studied in both individual and combined data analysis. The individual categories of post-partum depression, psychiatric problem (undifferentiated), stress, alcoholism, schizophrenia, and suicidal thought disturbance were all combined to create the category of total psychiatric diagnosis. The individual categories of physical handicap, arthritis, at home with undifferentiated illness, diabetes, cardiovascular disease, senility, lung disease, and cancer were all combined to create the category of total medical diagnoses. The individual categories of sick child with parent working, parentless home, and new baby were combined to create the total child care needs diagnostic category.

In the second area of category groupings, individual categories of undifferentiated personal care, ambulate, change dressings, help dress, help bathe, monitor health, assist with medication, and replace Home Care nurse became the total category of personal care practice. Care for children existed both as an individual as well as a total practice category. Individual categories of home care (undifferentiated), clean, do laundry, prepare meals, and shop were combined for the total practice category of housekeeping practice. Individual sub-categories were tabulated for the years 1976 and 1980. The combined categories were tabulated for 1976 vs. 1980 (total); 1976 vs. 1980 (excluding all LTC clients); and 1980 (LTC clients) vs. 1980 (non-LTC clients). The decision to combine the individual categories into combined, tabulated categories was based on the finding that most of the individual categories were not statistically significant, and in some cases were overlapping.

Individual Categories of Practice

The individual categories of the overall practice category displayed the following trends. Areas in which there was an increase in particular services being received by clients were: assistance with undifferentiated personal care; replacing the home care nurse temporarily; cleaning; preparing meals; and shopping. Decreases occurred in the areas of: assisting with dressing changes; caring for children; doing laundry; and housekeeping (undifferentiated). New categories were created in 1980 that did not exist in 1976. These were: monitoring the client's health status (e.g., noting changes in vital signs); assisting with medications (e.g., giving prepoured medication to the client); helping to ambulate; dress; and bathe.

Individual Categories of Diagnosis

In the area of individual client diagnosis, the area that refers specifically to the problems the client experiences as a precursor to needing homemaker assistance, the following trends were observed. Increases occurred in 1980 within the client diagnostic categories of: undifferentiated psychiatric problems; alcoholism; physical handicap; at home with undiagnosed illness; diabetic condition; cardiovascular disease; and cancer. Decreases occurred in the areas of: stress syndrome; arthritis; senility; lung disease; sick child with parent working; parentless home; and new baby.

The individual categories, while displaying interesting trends in practice and diagnosis, cannot be construed as being statistically significant. Given the diverse spread of categories, a decision was made to combine the individual subsets of diagnosis and practice into the more statistically accurate groupings of: total personal care practice, total child care practice, total housekeeping practice, total psychiatric diagnosis, total medical diagnosis, and total child care needs diagnosis. These specific, individual categories do not appear as such within the tabular format.

Quantitative Statements Concerning the Statistical Analysis

Sex of Client

The homemaker clients in this study were shown to be predominately female in both years; 87.9% in 1976; 79.0% in 1980.

Age of Client

The client of 1980 also increased in age with a significant increase occurring in those 80–90 years: 9.8% in 1976 compared to 25.9% in 1980. 47.2% of the LTC clients were aged 80–90 years. There was a corresponding decrease in 1980 of clients under the age of forty.

Number in Family Unit

The client of 1980 represented a smaller family unit. LTC clients were especially representative of decreased family units, with 68.4% living alone.

Method of Referral

It is important to note that the Long Term Care (LTC) division of the Ministry of Health did not exist in 1976. By 1980, following the creation of this LTC division in 1978, 43.3% of all clients to this homemaker agency were referred by the client or the client's relative; by 1980 this referral mode had decreased to only 3.3%.

Combined Practice Categories

When the above individual categories were combined for overall analysis, the following picture of homemaker practice appeared. Total personal care practice increased from 13.0% in 1976 to 42.0% in 1980. In 1980 56.4% of those receiving personal care assistance were LTC clients. Total child care practice decreased from 45.0% in 1976 to 19.0% in 1980, with no LTC clients receiving this service. Total housekeeping practice displayed no significant differentiation in the percentage of clients receiving this service in either year, with 93.0% of the clients in 1976 receiving housekeeping assistance, 97.0% in 1980. 92.3% clients receiving housekeeping service were LTC clients; 100% of the non-LTC clients had help with their housework.

Combined Diagnosis Categories

The combined category of diagnoses presents the following information about the homemaker client. Total psychiatric diagnosis increased from 8.0% of the clients in 1976 to 20.0% in 1980. In 1980 there were 27.9% of the non-LTC clients in this category, as opposed to 7.7% in the same year. Total medical diagnoses increased from 65.0% in 1976 to 80.0% in 1980. A higher percentage of LTC clients had a medical diagnosis problem, with 94.9% of all LTC clients having a medical diagnosis as opposed to 70.5% of the non-LTC clients. In total child care problems a decrease occurred with 28.0% of 1976 clients in this category, while 6.0% had this problem in 1980.

The Provus Discrepancy Model Applied to Homemakers

The Provus Discrepancy Model is a research mode that allows for a detailed, multi-stage analysis of the level of congruency or discrepancy that appears to exist between what the homemaker in this agency practiced and the theory that a majority of these homemakers had been taught. The curriculum of the homemaker program that was used in the discrepancy evaluation contains a series of seven tracks of teaching and student activities. They are: Track A (Orientation to Employment Market), Track B (Orientation to Occupational Role and Function), Track C (Protection in the Home), Track D (Nutrition), Track E (Growth and Development), Track F (Communications), and Track G (Health).

In preparing the data for this discrepancy evaluation phase, the total curriculum of the program was analyzed for comparative purposes with the statistical practice categories. The writer's intent was to determine where and to what extent a particular homemaker practice appeared to have been taught within the homemaker training program, 1980 format. The initial study contains a detailed analysis of the situation (Auman, 1981). For the purpose of this paper a summary of this analysis is provided.

Summarizing the results of the Provus Discrepancy analysis, it was found that congruency between theory and practice existed in eight of the eleven areas of practice. Congruency occurred in the practice/theory categories of: ambulate client, help dress, help bathe, care for children, clean, do laundry, prepare meals, and shop for groceries. Discrepancy between theory and practice occurred in the categories of: monitor health state, assist with medication, and replace homecare nurse temporarily.

DISCUSSION AND RECOMMENDATIONS

Change and Its Implications

Whereas, the client in 1980 differs significantly from her 1976 counterpart, it cannot be argued that this change is solely due to the creation of Long Term Care (LTC) in 1978. Clients with personal care needs in 1980 who were not associated with LTC increased significantly. The same is true for non-LTC clients in 1980 who experienced psychiatric as well as medical problems. Viewed as a whole, the homemaker situation appears to display a number of inherent problems. The inferences that can be drawn from the research are related specifically to the role, theory, and practice of the homemaker as it affected both the LTC and the non-LTC client.

The overall findings in this area were that the role of the homemaker has changed significantly between 1976 and 1980. The homemaker appears to have been placed in a situation in which increasing demands are being placed on her capacity to meet the rapidly changing needs of her client. Not only is her client older, having a notable degree of medical and psychiatric problems that often necessitate a myriad array of complex health care services, but this same client is part of a smaller family unit and may be more socially isolated than was her 1976 counterpart.

Role of the Homemaker as the "Good Samaritan"

One of the more intriguing aspects of the homemaker role is that of the homemaker as the "Good Samaritan" in her relationship with the client. The interviews conducted with the homemaker supervisors and the various notations that appear on sample client files appear to affirm this phenomenon as occurring with some regularity.

In the majority of the two hundred client case files that were read for the purpose of data analysis in this study, the homemaker appeared to be performing services for the client that could be described as housekeeping duties. For example, in the agency files she would frequently be described as being involved in: "helping Mrs. ____ do the weekly shopping"; "may need to also prepare a light lunch on some days." The areas in which there appears to be a problem for the homemaker, the homemaker agency, the homemaker program training division, and other concerned homemaker-oriented bodies appear to follow with some precision the exact outline of discrepancy that were found in the Provus analysis. These areas of concern fall into a broad category that could be referred to as special health care assistance and are the practice categories of: monitoring the state of health of the client; assisting the client with medication; and replacing Home Care nurses on a temporary basis. These same practice areas also constitute service categories in which the homemaker may be involved with the client in a situation where the "Good Samaritan" principle is operative.

This particular situation and the concerns created by these homemaker practices are found to be an often repeated theme in the interviews with the supervisors of the homemakers of this agency. For example, one of the supervisors in her comments regarding the role of the homemaker replied: ". . . sometimes homemakers are involved in basic nursing areas (that) she shouldn't be in . . . she doesn't have nursing training. Sometimes she has to take over for the Home Care Nurse because there aren't enough of these nurses to go around. Problems arise in a crisis in certain situations. They (the homemakers) are the only people who can help."

Interpretation of Theory and Practice of the Homemaker

As previously stated, the three areas of theory/practice discrepancy noted in this study involve the homemaker's assistance to certain clients in temporarily replacing the Home Care nurse, administering medications, and monitoring health states. An example of the homemaker as Home Care nurse substitute can be illustrated by a handicapped client with extensive skin lesions who required a bed bath. Home Care had been requested, but was not available. The homemaker was not trained to replace the Home Care nurse, but did so. In the second area, certain clients's charts indicated difficulty with self-administration of medication, and the homemaker was requested to assist them. In the area of monitoring health states a typical example was that of a client with cardiovascular problems who required monitoring the pulse rate related to medication usage. These three areas of practice are clearly outside the confines of the formal homemaker training program.

Interviews

Interviews with homemaker supervisors explored not only their interpretation of the homemaker role, but also their concerns about the congruence and discrepancy of homemaker practice and theory. In this area of theory and practice a majority of the supervisors prefaced their remarks by stating an awareness that in certain situations the homemaker may be providing services that do not match the theory taught by the homemaker program. However, in these instances, the supervisors frequently referred back to their statements regarding the "Good Samaritan" role of the homemaker. Only one of the four supervisors felt that the homemaker should receive formal training in these specific areas of discrepancy. For the majority, the feeling was that the present curriculum of the homemaker training program was more than adequate and that the homemaker should avoid taking on the role of a practical nurse or nurse's aide. An expansion of the service and client use of the Home Care nurse was seen as being the solution to the problem of homemaker practice that at times may be nursing rather than housekeeping.

CONCLUSIONS

It would appear that the homemaker, the agencies, the training programs, the Ministry of Health that purchases homemaker services, and last, but not least, the homemaker clients themselves are placed within an enigmatic situation. There is no simple, clear cut solution to the problem that now exists.

Viewing this complex situation of the homemaker's role, theory, and practice from a sociological point of view, the ownership of knowledge related especially to the area of personal care assistance, and also the corresponding control of that knowledge, appears to not be clearly established for all parties concerned (Berger and Luckman, 1966).

At the same time, with the dispersement of health and social service assistance to clients in home settings and away from the more rigidly controlled, institutional settings, such as hospitals, there may have occurred a corresponding loosening of previous areas of knowledge and practice control. That is to say that the nurse's aide, for example, within most hospital settings appears to have a rather well defined role. In most hospital settings there is a well defined and concisely executed control over the training program and the corresponding practice that this individual is expected to perform within the institution. For the homemaker within the research milieu of this study, these demarkations and control boundaries do not appear to have been established with the same precision as that of the aide in institutional settings. It would then appear that the dispersal of certain clients with health care needs into home rather than institutional settings carries with it specific problems as well as advantages, both to the client and the taxpayer.

The third issue that appears to be intertwined with this complex situation is the possibility that home care assistance may in certain situations not be the best solution for the client. There appears to have been, especially during the seventies, an understanding that home care was the ultimate answer to the problem of health and social service assistance to the chronically ill, the elderly, and the dependent individual. While this form of assistance is both cost beneficial and medically effective for some clients, it cannot be assumed that it is suitable for all. Given the paucity of any research related to the multiplicity of factors that must be considered in assessing this form of assistance, its widespread use without adequate research must be questioned.

The final issue that appears to be a continual problem for those involved in the homecare service area is the question of who is ultimately in control of this entity we refer to as homemakers. At present, without the existence of some form of licensure of the homemakers, their control boundaries are very ill defined. The levels of training of the homemakers vary widely throughout the province in which this study was conducted. Some of these homemakers have been trained by the community college homemaker programs. Others have only minimal on the job training. The client, it appears, has no assurance of uniformity of training. Indeed, the practice discrepancies that appear within this closely defined research area may be much more extensive for other agencies and their homemakers. This contemporary state of discrepancy will continue to exist until such time that there is some clearly established, uniform guidelines for all agencies, all training programs, and all homemakers practicing in the province.

RECOMMENDATIONS

Having studied the research findings related to the homemaker, the writer makes the following recommendations concerning the occupation of homemaking as it exists within the Province of British Columbia.

1. *It is recommended that the Ministry of Health, in consultation with all homemaker agencies and all homemaker training programs throughout the province, should establish clearcut guidelines for the role and practice of the homemaker that will be uniform in their usage by homemakers and strictly enforced throughout the province.* Additionally, that the Ministry of Health in the Province of British Columbia should assume the ultimate legal liability in the area of homemaker practice. Finally, within this area of homemaker practice there should be very close supervision of agencies and homemakers for the purpose of assuring optimal, safe levels of service to all clients.

2. *It is recommended that a process of licensing the home-*

maker be instituted. This act of licensing homemakers throughout the province would serve to assure the client that a homemaker, employed by any given agency within the province, would in fact have received adequate homemaker training and would possess the proper qualifications needed to meet specific client needs.

3. *In the area of training, it is recommended that the provincial and/or the federal government provide adequate educational funding assistance for homemakers already practicing who have not received formal training in homemaking.* Furthermore, these homemakers should be encouraged to upgrade their training levels by sustained support and encouragement of not only their agency employers but also by the provincial government that is the ultimate purchaser of their service.

4. *It is also recommended that the community colleges currently involved in the training of homemakers expand their educational expertise to make available in-service programs for all homemaker agencies within the province.*

5. *The final recommendation is that there be expanded and accelerated research within the broad area of homemaker concerns.* Given the rapidly changing dimensions of the homemaker's role and practice, it is imperative that decisions related to these areas, and indeed to the whole of homemaking as an occupational entity, be assisted by means of ongoing research and development.

REFERENCES

Auman, Jane. *An Evaluation of the Role, Theory, and Practice of the Occupation of Homemaker. Unpublished Master's Thesis,* The University of British Columbia, 1981.

Berger, Peter L. and Luckman, Thomas. *The Social Construction of Reality.* Garden City, New York: Doubleday and Company, 1966.

Canadian Council on Social Development. *Visiting Homemaker Services in Canada: Report of a Survey with Recommendations.* Prepared by the Advisory Committee on Visiting Homemaker Services, Ottawa, March, 1971.

Holsti, Ole. *Content Analysis for the Social Sciences and Humanities.* Don Mills, Ontario: Addison-Wesley Publishing Company, 1969.

MacIntyre, Sally. "Old Age as a Social Problem," in R. Dingwall (Ed.), *Health Care and Health Knowledge.* London: Croom Helm, Ltd., 1977.

Provus, Malcolm. *Discrepancy Evaluation.* Berkeley: McCutchan Publication Corporation, 1971.

Robinson, Nancy. *Costs of Homemaker—Home Health Aides,* 1974. ERIC Document Reproduction Service No. Ed. 107879.

Australia:
Special Needs
in Health Care—The Aged

Peter Sinnett, MD

ABSTRACT. Australian health and welfare services have developed in an ad hoc fashion. In response to demands by interested groups within the community, governments have relied on fiscal control and political expediency to regulate the growth of services and benefits. The lack of comprehensive policies and adequate planning has resulted in legislative complexity and administrative fragmentation, which has adversely affected the development of effective health and welfare services for the elderly Australian. The nature of these difficulties is discussed and recommendations are made for their resolution.

CURRENT SITUATION

It is estimated that in the financial year 1981–82 the Commonwealth Government spent in excess of 5.5 thousand million dollars on health and welfare programs designed principally for the care of the elderly. Of this sum 4.5 thousand million dollars or 82% of the total was spent on pensions and allowances, 11% on institutional care and 7% on community programs.

In spite of the fact that this expenditure represents 15–18% of total Commonwealth Government outlay, Australia lacks a clearly enunciated policy in relation to the care of the elderly, nor has the government the administrative mechanisms to ensure that expenditure is translated into effective service provision at the level of the community.

Peter Sinnett is Professor of Geriatrics, University of New South Wales, Geriatric Medicine Professorial Unit, St. George Hospital, Kogarah, New South Wales 2217, Australia.

This paper was presented at the Australian National University Conference on Health Policy, July 27–29, 1982.

It has been traditional in Australia for health and welfare services for the elderly to develop in an ad hoc fashion, largely as a result of demands by voluntary, private enterprise and professional groups involved in the provision of aged persons care. In response to demands by such groups governments have tended to rely heavily on fiscal control directed by political expediency to regulate the growth of services and benefits. This is unfortunate, as administration based on fiscal control of policy initiatives, generated by diverse and often self interested community groups gives no assurance that the resulting range of services will be balanced, comprehensive, equitable or cost effective.

THE IMPACT OF SOCIAL AND DEMOGRAPHIC CHANGE

Demographic and social changes within the Australian community will place pressure on governments to increase the efficiency of the health and welfare programs.

Ageing is associated with a marked increase in the prevalence of chronic illness and in the level of dependency. Some 27% of people aged between 65–74 years suffer from a chronic condition that limits their physical activity and independence. By contrast 42% of people over the age of 75 years are so affected. Hence any increase in the number of elderly people will be associated with an increase in the level of disability. Professor Pollard's[1] work indicates there is likely to be a 62% increase in the population over the age of 65 years between now and the turn of the century. Further the population aged 75–84 years will increase by 95% and the number of people over the age of 85 years will increase 190%. The implications for health care and welfare systems can be seen if we consider two separate diseases—dementia and fractures of the femoral neck.

The prevalence rate of dementia increases with increasing age from 3% in the 65–74 year age group to 26% in people over the age of 85 years. As a consequence we can anticipate that the number of persons suffering from moderate to severe dementia in Australia will increase from the present 96,000 to

---

[1]Pollard, A. H. (1982). "The Financing of Aged Care." *Australian Economic Trends,* No. 191. Published by Development Finance Corporation, Limited, Investment Bankers.

191,000 by the turn of the century and the number of nursing home beds required to care for these people will rise from 26,000 to a projected 52,000.

The same trend exists for fractures of the femoral neck. Here the incidence rate increases from 2.1/1000 in the 65–74 year age group to 26/1000 over the age of 85 years. At the present time some 8,300 elderly Australians fracture their femoral necks each year. By the turn of the century this figure will rise to 17,500 individuals and in consequence the number of acute hospital bed days required for the care of these people will rise from its present level of 287,000 to an estimated 604,000 by the year 2001.

While the demand for institutional, hospital and community care for the elderly is clearly going to increase between now and the turn of the century, the community's capacity to cope and care for its elderly is likely to decrease. Alterations in the Australian labour force of recent years is the basis for this prediction. Since 1966 elderly persons have been progressively displaced from the labour force. In 1966, 57.3% of males over the age of 55 years were in the labour force, by 1981 the level of participation by this group had fallen to 40.1%, a drop of 17.2%. Thus, based on 1966 employment levels, there are now 215,000 fewer men over the age of 55 in the workforce. Less marked reductions have occurred in the employment of elderly women. Overall the economic and social dependency of this age group has been clearly increased. By contrast over the same period there has been an increase in the order of 50% in the participation rate in the work force for women aged between 25–44 years. Thus the family's capacity to undertake long-term care for the elderly has been reduced.

The projected increase in the demand for aged persons' services coupled with the anticipated decrease in the family's capacity to provide such care will increase the financial burden on government. Faced with this increased burden it would seem essential for government to develop an overall policy for the care of the elderly Australian so that priorities for expenditure can be developed on a rational basis. At the same time it is essential that government develop administrative mechanisms to ensure that expenditure is translated into effective service provision at the level of the community.

REQUIREMENTS FOR EFFECTIVE AGED PERSONS SERVICES

In addition to the provision of an adequate income maintenance scheme indexed to the cost of living, the effective care of the elderly depends upon the provision of an integrated range of community, hospital-based and institutional services organised on a regional basis. (A suggested list of such services is presented in Appendix 1.)

It is stressed that the service components in aged persons' care are in large measure interdependent, so that a deficiency in one area will be associated with inappropriate use of a related facility. Thus, if home nursing services and home laundry services are deficient, it is highly likely that an incontinent patient will be placed in a nursing home. Similarly, if an acute hospital is unable to admit a patient with transient ischaemic episodes, it is highly likely that following a stroke this patient will be admitted to an institution.

There is real danger in times of economic restraint that governments may be tempted to place restrictions on the provision of relatively expensive hospital and institutional facilities on the assumption that community services are a viable alternative. Of course, the truth of the matter is that these services are complementary and are not necessarily true alternatives. Irrespective of the level of community services, the need for institutional care increases with age. It therefore follows that any policy which selectively develops community programs, while at the same time restricting hospital and institutional services, runs the risk of transferring resources from areas of greater to areas of lesser need and of selectively disadvantaging those elderly people with the greatest burden of physical and intellectual dependency.

While geriatric services must be community oriented and include both adequate domiciliary and rehabilitation facilities, they must have above all else a strong clinical base in an acute regional hospital. Second grade geriatric hospitals which are often little more than ghettos and which will serve to deny the elderly access to facilities readily available to other age groups in our community must be avoided at all costs.

It is only when specialist geriatric services with access to adequate diagnostic facilities and staffing levels are accepted as an integral component of university teaching hospitals that the standard of care offered the elderly Australian will start to approach that offered to younger age groups in our community. Such a development is essential if doctors and other health professionals are to be adequately trained in the care of the aged and chronically ill.

Finally, it is only when adequate hospital-based geriatric services are provided that we can expect essential clinical research to be undertaken into such fundamental questions as the nature of the ageing process and its physiological consequences as well as into such important causes of disability and dependency as acute confusional states, and altered drug reactions among the elderly and the mechanism of falls and fractures among the aged. Without such research it is difficult to see how the quality of life of the elderly Australian is to be significantly improved.

DEFICIENCIES IN AGED PERSONS SERVICES

Unfortunately, in spite of high levels of government expenditure many communities in Australia do not have access to a comprehensive geriatric service, and it is well known that the standards of care for aged people varies markedly, not only throughout Australia but within separate states of the Commonwealth. Three difficulties are common:

1. An absolute deficiency in an essential component of the geriatric service.
2. Lack of co-ordination between service components, often the result of fragmentation in service delivery between government, private enterprise and voluntary agencies.
3. The level of service provision often does not parallel social need. This situation is illustrated in three diagrams[2] which relate the provision of nursing home accommodation, pensioner housing and day centres to social need within one of Sydney's Metropolitan Health Regions. As can be seen, nursing home provision is negatively related to need. Provision of Housing Commission units is positively related while the provision of day centres bears no relationship to social need.

---

[2]Sinnett, Peter, based on unpublished data from study, commissioned by Auditor-General, on behalf of Australian Government.

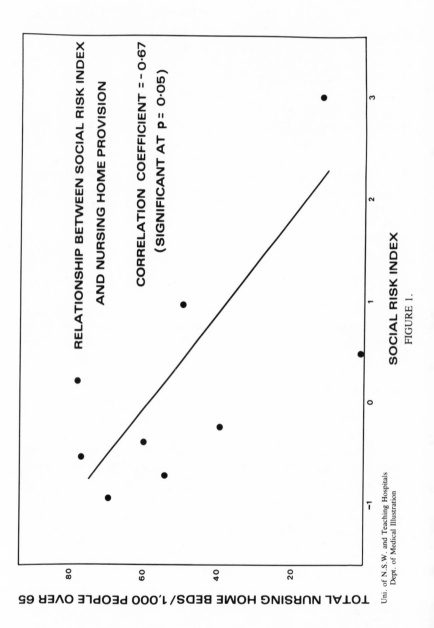

RELATIONSHIP BETWEEN SOCIAL RISK INDEX
AND NURSING HOME PROVISION

CORRELATION COEFFICIENT = - 0·67
(SIGNIFICANT AT p= 0·05)

SOCIAL RISK INDEX

FIGURE 1.

TOTAL NURSING HOME BEDS / 1,000 PEOPLE OVER 65

Uni. of N.S.W. and Teaching Hospitals
Dept. of Medical Illustration

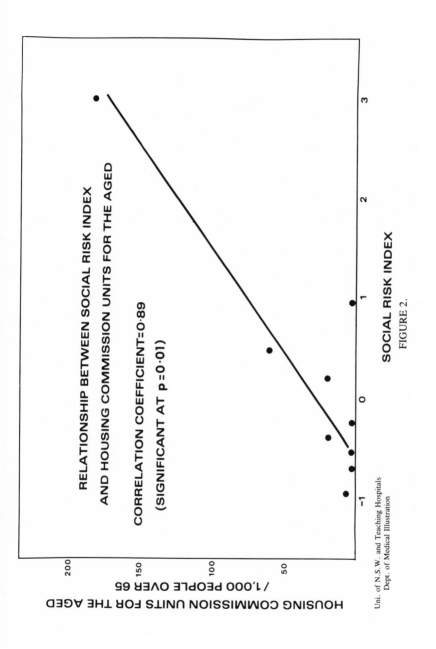

RELATIONSHIP BETWEEN SOCIAL RISK INDEX
AND HOUSING COMMISSION UNITS FOR THE AGED

CORRELATION COEFFICIENT=0·89

(SIGNIFICANT AT p=0·01)

HOUSING COMMISSION UNITS FOR THE AGED
/ 1,000 PEOPLE OVER 65

SOCIAL RISK INDEX

FIGURE 2.

Uni. of N.S.W. and Teaching Hospitals
Dept. of Medical Illustration

165

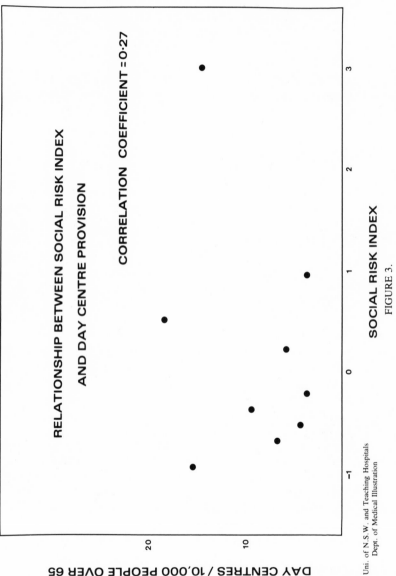

RELATIONSHIP BETWEEN SOCIAL RISK INDEX
AND DAY CENTRE PROVISION

CORRELATION COEFFICIENT = 0·27

SOCIAL RISK INDEX

FIGURE 3.

DAY CENTRES / 10,000 PEOPLE OVER 65

LEGISLATIVE AND ADMINISTRATIVE DIFFICULTIES INHIBITING THE DEVELOPMENT OF HEALTH AND WELFARE SERVICES FOR THE ELDERLY

Legislative and administrative difficulties contribute significantly to deficiencies in the delivery of geriatric services.

The random growth of health and welfare services for the elderly is responsible for the large body of poorly co-ordinated Commonwealth and State legislation which controls the use of funds for the aged persons' programs. Thus nursing home proposals compete against each other for funds under the Aged or Disabled Persons Homes Act. Hostels proposals compete against each other for funds provided under both the Aged Persons Hostels act and the Aged or Disabled Persons Homes Act. Independent living units may be funded by either the Housing Assistance Act Part III or the Aged or Disabled Persons Homes Act. Community programs compete against community programs for funds provided under the States Grants (Home Care) Act, the Delivered Meals Subsidy Act, the Aged or Disabled Persons Homes Act and the National Health Act. Hospital based geriatric services now depend for funds on State Governments. Destitute elderly are provided for under the Homeless Persons Assistance Act. Elderly returned service personnel are supported by a separate range of legislation administered by the Department of Veteran's Affairs. Finally income maintenance schemes for the elderly are funded under the Social Services Act.

The body of legislation that comprises the Commonwealth Government's health and welfare programs for the elderly is administered separately at the Federal level by three autonomous departments, Social Security, Health and Veteran's Affairs. Thus administrative complexity is added to legislative fragmentation. Nowhere is there an overview which would enable assessment of aged persons' services and their funding arrangements. Of necessity decisions are taken in isolation by the various departments without full awareness of their impact on the efficiency and cost structure of the overall program. The absence of a single body responsible for the coordination of aged persons' programs has adversely affected program planning, program implementation and program evaluation and control.

A further difficulty arises from the fact that there is no one-to-one relationship between legislation and service provision. A given service is often funded under more than one Act. As an example, Home Nursing Services with the (former) Southern Metropolitan Health Region of New South Wales are funded under three separate instruments.

The Sydney Home Nursing Service is treated as a Schedule 4 hospital. The Rockdale Community Nursing Service, the Kogarah Community Nursing Service and the Hurstville Home Nursing Service are each funded under the Home Subsidy Act, Home Nursing carried out by the staff of the New South Wales Health Commission is supported by the Commonwealth Government under the Community Health Program. Hence it is extremely unlikely that the Commonwealth Government is fully aware of the extent to which it is supporting home nursing services in this health region. In consequence, it would be difficult for the government to respond adequately to requests for additional funds for nursing services or to defend the present level of support for nursing services in this region. The capacity of governments to respond appropriately to requests for incresed services is further weakened by the absence of agreed statutory "norms" which would serve as a basis for the regulation of the supply of services on a regional basis.

Further complexities arise at the level of Commonwealth/ State/Local Government co-ordination. In the case of nursing homes, approval for new accommodation is recommended by the Commonwealth/State Co-ordinating Committee on Nursing Homes. Regional need is measured against an arbitrary norm of 50 nursing home beds/1000 of the population over the age of 65 years. The Commonwealth Government approves homes for purposes of Commonwealth funding (benefits or deficit funding) but the nursing home is licensed by the State Health Authority. In the case of other forms of aged persons' accommodation approval of new facilities does not at present require the recommendation of a Commonwealth/State or local Co-ordinating Committee and there is no agreed norm to regulate the level of service provision. Further, in New South Wales licensing of hostels is the responsibility of the State Department of Youth & Community Services.

MAJOR PROBLEMS IDENTIFIED

1. Absence of a single body within the Commonwealth Government charged with the responsibility of co-ordinating programs and monitoring expenditure on aged persons' services.
2. Relevant legislation is administered independently by three autonomous Commonwealth Government departments.
3. Many aged persons' services are funded under more than one Act.
4. Lack of comprehensive aged persons' care programs organised on a regional basis.
5. Lack of statutory "norms" to regulate the level of service provision on a regional basis.
6. Lack of agreement between government departments as to a suitable demographic unit to serve as a basis for accounting and service provision.
7. Interdependence of geriatric services is not considered when funds are allocated.
8. Lack of adequate Commonwealth/State/Local Government co-ordination of services. Nursing homes are reviewed by a Commonwealth/State Co-ordinating Committee on Nursing Homes. However, a similar committee does not exist for the review of other forms of accommodation or indeed for the review of any of the other aged persons' services funded by the Commonwealth.
9. Lack of standard licensing requirements for aged persons' accommodation.
10. Lack of adequate assessment procedures for admission to aged persons' accommodation.
11. Lack of Commonwealth Government initiative in determining location of Nursing Homes and other forms of accommodation. Geographic distribution of facilities is left to the initiative of the applicant.

12. Lack of hospital based services specialising in the assessment, treatment and rehabilitation of geriatric patients.

GENERAL RECOMMENDATIONS

1. Define a demographic unit, such as the State Health Region, which will provide all relevant Commonwealth Government departments with a common basis for the financing of services and for accounting procedures.
2. Define the range of services considered essential for the adequate care of the elderly in our community and support funding of these services. Commonwealth financial support will thereby be translated into a comprehensive and integrated program of aged persons' care organised on a regional basis.
3. Establish statutory "norms" to regulate the level of service provision required to provide an adequate program of aged persons' care organised on a regional basis.
4. Establish on a regional basis a register of services, including those funded both directly and indirectly by the Commonwealth Government. Services registered should be classified according to function, i.e., income maintenance programs, day centres, home nursing services, nursing home accommodation, etc. The register would enable the Commonwealth to relate the level of service provision and thus to undertake service evaluation.
5. Establish an interdepartmental committee of the Commonwealth Government charged with the responsibility of co-ordinating information on a regional basis as to the level of funding and service provision in the area of aged persons' care. The maintenance of regional funding and service registers should be the responsibility of this committee. The integrated regional information would be supplied to relevant Commonwealth Government departments with advice as to areas in which funding was either above or below the level required to meet agreed "norms" of service provision.

Information would also be supplied to Commonwealth/ State Co-ordinating Committees to assist them in formulating advice to appropriate Commonwealth and State Ministers.

6. Expand the role of the Commonwealth/State Co-ordinating Committees on Nursing Homes initially to include the development of recommendations on all forms of aged persons' accommodation. Later this role should be expanded to include recommendations on all regionally based aged persons' services. This would ensure that Commonwealth and State Governments received uniform advice and that a balanced program of community, hospital and institutional services resulted.
7. Establish a working party to advise on possible rationalisation of aged persons' health and welfare legislation.
8. Establish standard licensing procedures for all forms of subsidised aged persons' accommodation.
9. Establish adequate assessment procedures for admission to all forms of subsidised aged persons' accommodation.
10. Establish architectural guidelines to be adhered to in the construction of all new nursing homes.
11. Extend the range of the extensive care nursing home benefit to include patients requiring constant supervision due to intellectual impairment.
12. Encourage the establishment of hospital based geriatric services specialising in the assessment, treatment and rehabilitation of geriatric patients.

APPENDIX 1

RANGE OF GERIATRIC SERVICES

I. Community Services

1. Council employed Social Workers/Welfare Officers.
2. Community Information Service.
3. Home Visiting Service.

4. Home Maintenance Program.
5. Home Surveillance Program.
6. Home Help Service.
7. Delivered Meals Service.
8. Home Laundry Service.
9. Senior Citizens Clubs.
10. Day Centres.
11. General Practitioners with access to the range of services.
12. Home Nursing Service—with 24 hour emergency cover.
13. Community Health Centres.
14. Extended Care Service—with facilities to arrange equipment loans and the capacity to organise necessary home modifications.
15. Transport Services.

II. Hospital Services

1. Day Hospitals.
2. Geriatric Outpatients Departments.
3. Community Liaison Sisters—to assist hospitals with discharge planning.
4. Geriatric Medical Unit—for treatment and assessment.
5. Crisis admission beds—for emergency social admissions from community.
6. Psychogeriatric Unit.

III. Institutional Services and Accommodation

1. Housing Commission Units.
2. Self Contained Accommodation.
3. Holiday Relief Accommodation.
4. Hostel Accommodation.
5. Nursing Home Accommodation.
6. Hospice for the Dying.

APPENDIX 2

SERVICE DEFICIENCIES

1. Home Maintenance Programs
2. Home Surveillance Programs.
3. Home Laundry Services.
4. 24 Hour Emergency Nursing Care.
5. Extended Care Services.
6. Transport Services.
7. Day Hospitals.
8. Geriatric Outpatients Departments.
9. Hospital Based Community Liaison Sisters.
10. Geriatric Medical Units.
11. Crisis Admission Beds.
12. Psychogeriatric Units.

Home Support Services in Australia: A Confusion of Intergovernmental Responsibilities and Provision

Elizabeth M. Coombs, BA (Hons) Psych., CPhil

ABSTRACT. This article describes the current provision of community and domiciliary health and welfare services in Australia focusing upon national programs and outlining how these have been interpreted and implemented by each of the six States and two Territories which constitute the Australian Federation. The funding of home support services is described, particularly in relation to institutional services and State differences. Changing emphases have been highlighted and considered relative to the needs of those requiring support to remain at home. The article presents an account of a medley of initiatives and programs which are failing to meet ever increasing demand.

The recent report of an Inquiry into Accommodation and Home Care for the Aged and the policy of the recently elected Australian Labor Party in relation to domiciliary care are examined.

Although historically home support services were introduced in Australia to meet the needs of broadly defined groups such as 'the poor and the sick', the present day users and the group to whom legislation underpinning these services is primarily directed, are elderly Australians. Indeed, this group is by far the greatest consumer of community and domiciliary services. In the context of the recent awareness of changing demographic trends and the increasing representation of the aged in the world's population, the above situa-

Elizabeth M. Coombs is Research and Resource Analyst with the Home Care Service of New South Wales, Sydney, Australia. She has an Honours degree in Psychology and is currently undertaking a doctoral thesis on domiciliary support services for the chronically ill and disabled at the School of Health Administration, University of New South Wales, Sydney, Australia.

tion would appear to be the result of sensitive and successful long-term planning. Unfortunately not. Care of the aged and the provision of non-institutional services has been a low priority on the Australian health and welfare agenda. Awareness of the 'ageing' of Australia's population and the high cost of institutional care has produced a new emphasis and sudden attention is now being directed towards the ad hoc, fragmented and unco-cordinated services which maintain the elderly and other people in their own homes.

It is the aim of this article to provide an overview of home support services in Australia. First, however, some terminology. There are a plethora of terms, phrases and definitions used to delineate the various programs and services which all have in common the fact that they are not delivered in an institution. Many of them, however, are based at institutional facilities such as hospitals. 'Non-institutional' care in this article is used to describe those services which do not require the user to reside at the same location as the services to obtain their use. This broad group of non-institutional services in Australia has two main forms: community and domiciliary services. Domiciliary services are those health and welfare services which go to the consumer in their own homes, while the term 'community services' is used to describe those services which bring the users to an activity or service that is situated outside their own homes without requiring them to reside at the service origin.

In 1982/83 the Australian Government will spend approximately $Aust.960 million on accommodation and home care for the aged. Of this $890 million will be spent on residential accommodation and care, while $70 million (7%) shall be spent upon home support services such as home nursing, home help and delivered meals. Despite lip service to the concept of providing the chronically ill and disabled with the means to live in their own home, the gross disparity between institutional and non-institutional provisions has grown rather than diminished over the years. Since 1976/77, the expenditure on institutional care has increased by over $565 million. In contrast, expenditure on community and domiciliary programs has increased by only $45 million. Furthermore, expenditure on institutional care was nine times greater than expenditure on home care in 1976/77 but had grown to eleven times greater than home care expenditure by 1982/83 (Macleay, 1982).

To understand the Australian provision of health and welfare services, it is necessary to remember that Australia is a federation of States with three levels of government. The Federal or Commonwealth Government has powers and duties under the Constitution to provide certain programs. However, it is limited in its ability to directly provide health services. The Federal Government, by legislation, can provide funds to organisations, statutory authorities and other levels of government to provide these services. Thus the mechanism for determining and allocating public financial support for health and welfare services is dispersed among Federal, State and local government sectors, religious and charitable organisations, individuals and private commercial interests. Funding arrangements between programs are also diverse; some programs are fully Federally funded, others are cost shared according to a variety of arrangements. Further, while the Commonwealth Government provides grants and the legislative framework for services, the State Governments are primarily responsible for the administration and the provision of some health, welfare and housing services and for the allocation of some Commonwealth funds to local governments and voluntary agencies. Thus there is a division of responsibility for the paying benefits and subsidies on one hand and the administration and regulation on the other. This situation has worked against home support services as the Federal government alone pays benefits to nursing home patients and assists with the funding of non profit nursing homes. As the State Governments contribute to the cost of home health and welfare services and not to nursing home costs, there has been no financial incentive for State Governments to develop comprehensive community and domiciliary services. On the contrary, there have been definite disincentives.

Some Commonwealth legislation makes provision for the Federal Government to provide funds directly to local government. However, local government involvement in health and welfare is minimal, particularly in the State of New South Wales (NSW). Henderson and Lewis (1980) calculated the comparative personal and community services expenditure of State and local governments to be 95%–96% and 4%–5%

respectively. The traditional role of local government has been almost exclusively confined to services to property. The State Governments provide the wide range of education, health and social welfare functions carried out by local authorities in Great Britain and many other countries. There are enormous differences however, between and within States in local council involvement with domiciliary and community services. In Victoria, for example, local government plays a much greater role in direct service provision than in NSW. Victoria is the only State where home help, handyman and delivered meal services are provided or co-ordinated in any uniform and substantial way by local government authorities. Here 211 of the total 212 local councils directly provide home help services. In a seeming contradiction to the above assertion, only NSW Local Government Authorities provide home nursing services. In this State seventeen local governments provide nursing care for a predominantly aged client group.

The lack of local government involvement in home support services across Australia is not due to limited eligibility for Commonwealth funds. On the contrary, local government authorities are eligible for Commonwealth funds for the provision of senior citizen centres, home care, paramedical services, home nursing and delivered meals as well as nursing homes and hostels. But for historical reasons, local council involvement in these services has been very limited.

COMMONWEALTH LEGISLATION AND PROGRAMS FOR DOMICILIARY AND COMMUNITY SUPPORT

There are a number of Commonwealth and State Acts which specifically relate to the provision of domiciliary and community services. Although emphasis within this article is placed upon the Commonwealth legislation as this is common to all States, within each State there are Acts and policies which further provide for those requiring long-term care. Sometimes these interact with programs provided at the Commonwealth level. In some cases, legislation that applies to institutional services, accommodation, etc. has sections that impinge upon the provision of domiciliary and community services. There is not room here to cover all the legislation of all States that have implications for the services under discussion.

The Commonwealth Departments involved with home support services are the Departments of Health, Social Security and Veterans' Affairs. Within each State there are a further two or three departments which administer the following programs and legislation: the Home Nursing Subsidy Act (1956); the States Grants (Paramedical Services) Act (1969); Delivered Meals Subsidy Act (1970); Domiciliary Nursing Care Benefit (1972); Handicapped Children's Allowances (1975) and the Community Health Program. Under this legislation, expenditure upon home nursing, 'home care', the Domiciliary Nursing Care Benefit and the Handicapped Children's Allowance, shall comprise 87% of the total expenditure estimated to be spent on the 1982/83 budget upon home support services. The payments made for all these programs in 1981/82 totalled $40 million. The payments made to each State for each program relative to the total, as well as the aged and invalid, population in each State has been detailed in Table 1. From this table it is apparent that the States in which to reside if one is elderly and/or an invalid, are Tasmania and Victoria.

HOME NURSING

The Home Nursing Subsidy Act (1956) was the first step taken by the Commonwealth Government to provide nursing care for the aged and disabled in their own homes. It was designed to assist in the extension of home nursing activities, either by expansion of organisations or by the formation of new ones. To receive subsidy, a home nursing service must be non-profit making, employ registered nurses and receive assistance from a State Government, a local government body or other authority established under a State Act.

Six States participate under this Act and considerable variation can be found between the States in the management, funding level, number of organisations, services available and patient populations of the home nursing services. Table 2 sets out the number of organisations, visits and staffing establishments for each State 1980/81.

In Western Australia the major organisation—the Silver

TABLE 1: COMMONWEALTH EXPENDITURE ON HOME SUPPORT SERVICES FOR EACH STATE, EXPENDITURE PER THE AGED AND INVALID POPULATION 1981/82*

State	Total '81 Aged & Invalid Pop'n	Delivered Meals Subsidy $	Per Aged & Invalid	States Grants (Home Care) Act $	Per Aged & Invalid	Home Nursing Subsidy $	Per Aged & Invalid	Domestic Nursing Care Benefit	Per Aged & Invalid
N.S.W.	666,445	1,227,056	1.84	6,148,409	9.23	3,467,042	5.20	7,176	0.01
Victoria	494,657	1,583,917	3.20	5,471,357	11.06	5,030,224	10.17	5,116	0.01
Qld.	315,615	451,598	1.43	2,330,187	7.38	3,378,798	10.71	3,985	0.01
S. Aust.	180,866	406,202	2.24	1,753,662	9.69	1,555,704	8.60	1,760	0.01
W. Aust.	148,756	422,302	2.83	1,457,480	9.80	2,848,469	19.15	1,769	0.01
Tasmania	53,353	136,996	2.56	911,241	17.08	510,867	9.58	1,365	0.03
N.T.	5,880	6,499	1.11	b	b	b	b	a	a
A.C.T.	14,136	18,218	1.29	b	b	b	b	a	a
AUSTRALIA	1,879,708	4,252,788	2.26	18,072,336	9.84	16,791,104	8.93	21,172	

* Aged has been taken as when a person becomes eligible for the Aged Pension i.e. 60 years for women and 65 for men.

(a) Expenditure for the Northern Territory and A.C.T. included in expenditure for South Australia and New South Wales respectively.

(b) Non-participating States

Source: Annual Report of Commonwealth Department of Social Security, 1981/82.
Annual Report of Director-General of Health 1981/82.
Australian Bureau of Statistics, 1981 Census of Population and Housing, 1982.
Commonwealth Department of Health.

TABLE 2:   HOME NURSING ORGANISATIONS WITHIN AUSTRALIA,
             NURSING ESTABLISHMENTS, NUMBER OF PATIENTS,
             VISITS AND KILOMETRES TRAVELLED 1980/81

State	No. of Organizations	No. of Patients Treated	No. of Visits	No. of Nurses	No. of Kilometres	Amount $
New South Wales	90	82,697	1,376,039	429	4,742,364	2,947,832
Victoria	69	85,864	1,444,403	498	5,112,462	2,929,176
Queensland	9	10,608	377,458	445	1,466,754	2,616,584
W. Australia	2	34,921	867,789	260	3,449,103	2,309,422
Tasmania	20	12,012	213,818	65	808,639	368,942
Sth. Australia	1	11,889	449,498	198	1,982,721	1,316,803
	192	238,001	4,729,448	1,995	17,662,143	13,498,859

Source: Commonwealth Department of Health.

Chain Nursing Association—provides the widest range of services, such as nursing home beds, home help aides and 'substitute relative' aides, as well as home nursing services. Although the Blue Nursing Service (Queensland) also provides nursing home accommodation, the Royal District Nursing Service (Victoria) is the only other non-hospital based service which provides home health aides. Both of the largest home nursing services in Queensland and Victoria received funding under the Community Health Program (1973) which allowed them to establish comprehensive community nursing education programs.

It was estimated in the 1982/83 Federal Budget that expenditure under the Home Nursing Subsidy Act would total $21 million. As the wording of the Act stipulates that the Federal contribution cannot exceed that of the States, and as the State Governments differ in their willingness to support these nursing services, many of the home nursing organisations rely heavily upon community support which can vary from virtually nothing to over 25% of total funds.

Unfortunately, the most recent national surveys of domiciliary nursing organisations and their patients were completed in 1972 and 1974 respectively. These revealed that two-thirds of the organisations (n = 145) were hospital based and one-third non-hospital based. The latter group, however, treated 80% of all patients in the survey. Of the patients treated by non-hospital based services, five major organisations, one in each State except Tasmania, provided services to approximately 64% of patients. The latter survey revealed that 78% of the patient caseload was over the age of 65 years and that this proportion was relatively uniform across all States and all services. Other findings were that female patients outnumbered males by two to one; that heart and circulatory complaints are the major illnesses treated (29%) and that of patients receiving domiciliary nursing care, 51% received general nursing care and 20% supportive care.

DOMICILIARY AND COMMUNITY WELFARE

Housekeeping, senior citizen centres and welfare officers for the aged are provided by the State Grants (Home Care) Act (1969). Housekeeping or other forms of domestic assistance are stipulated to be provided wholly or mainly for aged persons. Initially funding was on a $1 to $1 basis, that is, equal funding by Commonwealth and State bodies. In 1973, the then Commonwealth Government (the Australian Labor Party) provided $2 to every $1 provided by the State Governments. This reverted in 1978 (under the Liberal Party) to $1:$1 arrangement for home care services and welfare officers while senior citizen centres remained at the $2:$1 level. Table 3 sets out expenditure allocation between home help, senior citizen centres and welfare officer programs.

As can be seen, domestic assistance has received the largest allocation since the Act's inception. During the last fourteen years the proportion allocated to it has increased while the amount provided for Senior Citizens' Centres has declined. There has been a growth also in the relative allocation to the welfare officer program. Changes in the relative allocations cannot be interpreted as due to shifts in policy. Rather, the differing nature of the recurring expenses involved with the home help services and welfare officers as compared to the largely capital outlay for the Senior Citizen Centres is more likely to have produced the shift noted above.

TABLE 3:   TOTAL EXPENDITURE AND PROPORTIONAL ALLOCATION
OF STATES GRANTS (HOME CARE) ACT, 1969/70 TO 1981/82*

Year	Home Services %	Senior Citizen Centres %	Welfare Officers %	Total Expenditure $
1969/70	66	33	1	47,850
1970/71*)) 1971/72*)	69	30	1	1,175,873
1972/73	54	44	2	1,686,614
1973/74	63	34	4	1,942,898
1974/75	67	26	7	4,615,790
1975/76	57	36	7	9,877,030
1976/77	60	35	5	11,557,996
1977/78	66	29	5	13,805,368
1978/79	69	24	7	12,458,013
1979/80	71	22	7	14,668,015
1980/81	69	24	7	16,761,611
1981/82	72	22	6	18,072,336
TOTAL				106,669,542

*   Only combined figures for 1970/71 and 1971/72 available.

Source: Annual Reports of Commonwealth Department of Social Security,
1969/70 to 1982/82.

Table 4 provides further detail of funding changes over time within each of the three programs and of the total expenditure. It can be easily seen from this Table how the Federal Government of the time effectively reduced their commitment to these programs by reducing the Federal contribution from 75% to 50%. From a period of massive expansion in 1974/75 and 1975/76 (138% and 114% increase in total expenditure respectively) percentage expenditure increases under this Act have steadily decreased. The present increase from the previous year is below the current inflation rate.

The policy underpinning the States Grants (Home Care) Act (1969) was to utilise the voluntary sector and organise voluntary action to operate home care services that aim to

TABLE 4:   STATES GRANTS (HOME CARE) ACT, FUNDING BY PROGRAM
             AND TOTAL EXPENDITURE, PERCENTAGE CHANGE 1969/70 TO 1981/82*

Year	Home Services		Senior Citizen Centres		Welfare Officers		Total	
	$	% Change	$	% Change	$	% Change	$	% Change
1969/70	31,413		16,000		437		47,850	
1970/71) 1971/72)	808,525		352,637		14,711		1,175,873	
1972/73	915,928		736,387		34,289		1,686,614	
1973/74	1,218,068	33	650,628	-12	74,202	116	1,942,898	+15
1974/75	3,099,754	154	1,196,756	84	319,280	103	4,615,790	+138
1975/76	5,668,376	45	3,560,692	198	648,030	103	9,877,030	+114
1976/77	6,891,077	22	3,996,839	12	670,080	30	11,557,996	+17
1977/78	9,137,848	33	3,946,196	-1	721,324	8	13,805,368	+19
1978/79	8,585,615	-6	3,050,323	-23	822,075	14	12,458,013	-10
1979/80	10,368,984	21	3,245,358	6	1,053,673	28	14,668,015	+18
1980/81	11,507,700	11	4,000,000	23	1,253,911	19	16,761,611	+14
1981/82	12,673,000	10	3,999,999	0	1,399,337	12	18,072,336	+8
TOTALS	70,906,288		28,751,905		7,011,349		106,669,542	

*   Only combined figures for the years 1970/71 and 1971/72 are available. Percentage yearly
       changes for these early years cannot be calculated.

Source: Annual Reports of Commonwealth Department of Social Security, 1969/70 to 1981/82.

assist those wishing to remain in their home or those who have no alternative, and who, as a result, need supportive or preventive services; and, to prevent the inappropriate institutionalisation of citizens. In most States this Act is administered by Departments of Health. However, in NSW, South Australia and Tasmania, administration of the Act is performed by Community Welfare departments. In NSW this responsibility is shared with the Department of Local Government which administers Senior Citizen Centres. Applications received by the State departments are recommended to the Department of Social Security for payment of subsidy. Eligible organisations include State, local government and community welfare bodies.

'Housekeeping or other domestic assistance' includes, in NSW, the cooking of meals within the client's home; general housekeeping; live-in relief services; personal care; homemakers; handyman and gardening services. There are considerable interstate differences, for example, South Australia and Tasmania include paramedical services such as chiropody and physiotherapy under home care while Victoria's Home Help Service does not provide assistance with minor household repairs. In Victoria from 20% to 30% of the services are provided for younger persons and families. This includes provision for live-in staff. In addition, a special State funded service is available for the care of the physically handicapped or mentally retarded clients. In one quarter of 1979, 1,543 mentally retarded and 513 physically handicapped clients were under care. The majority of these clients were children as eligibility is restricted to those whose disabilities were diagnosed before the age of eighteen years. NSW Home Care Service also has a special project designed to assist the disabled which receives joint State and Commonwealth funding.

In Queensland the provision of the service is governed by a means test. The Advisory Committee to the Queensland Department of Health on the care of the aged (1981) reports that service-wide utilisation data are not kept but that "enquiry of the two oldest metropolitan community health centres reveals that the average provision of home help is 1-1/4 to 1-1/2 hours per week. This is, as often as not, supplied two-weekly, and six hours per week is the maximum received by any client, though this amount is a rarity."

NSW is the only State which maintains detailed statistics of home help operations. A recent report (Coombs, 1983) stated that the hours of weekly service have steadily decreased from 2.5 in September 1980 to 1.3 hours in February 1983. In particular, the State's hospital rationalisation program has had enormous implications for the service through its reduction in hospital bed numbers and length of stay. The report concluded that increasing pressure is being put on the Home Care Service of NSW through increasing numbers of clients; greater needs of clients; a 'no-growth' budget and a decrease in hours provided free of charge by other organisations. The inability of the Service to meet these demands was said to be manifested in a decrease in the number of hours of service provided to each client each week, huge increases in the numbers of households refused services (2,150%) or given restricted services (313%) and an increase in the unpaid work performed by Home Care employees.

The Commonwealth Government subsidises State and local government expenditure on senior citizens' centres. This subsidy is paid on a $2:$1 basis, up to two-thirds of the capital costs. Commonwealth assistance is available also for furnishings, recreational facilities or forms of transport, provided such equipment is used in connection with the centre. A meals on wheels kitchen and equipment within a centre may also be funded. Services such as meals on wheels, podiatry, general counselling, domestic assistance and emergency transport may also be organised or co-ordinated from the centres. Although the centres and their facilities may be utilised by other organisations or groups, it is stipulated that the senior citizens must have priority. This priority and other factors have produced severe criticism of the program.

Since 1969, $20 million has been provided by the Federal Government under the Senior Citizens section of the Act. Like the services discussed earlier, there is considerable variation between States in the funding received for this program and in the number of centres established, particularly as a ratio to the number of aged persons living at home (Table 5).

Queensland and NSW have the highest ratio of population to centres (approximately one centre per 4,500 aged persons at home). Although they receive considerably different allocations, there is a significant drop to the ratio enjoyed by the

TABLE 5:   SUBSIDISED SENIOR CITIZENS CENTRES, BY STATE,
         % ALLOCATION, % AGED POPULATION AND RATIO OF CENTRES
                TO AGED POPULATION AT HOME, 1981/82

State	% of Funding Allocation	% of Aged pop'n	Number of Centres	Ratio of Centres To Aged Pop'n
New South Wales	28.8	35.4	115	1:4,243
Victoria	37.2	26.3	214	1:1,665
Queensland	10.6	16.8	45	1:4,716
South Australia	9.6	9.6	106	1:1,178
West Australia	9.9	7.9	48	1:2,110
Tasmania	3.3	2.8	17	1:2,235
Northern Territory	0.2	0.3	4	1: 850
Australian Capital Territory	0.4	0.8	3	1:2,367
TOTAL	100.0	100.0	552	

Source: Australian Census, 1981.
         Department of Social Security, Annual Report, 1981/82.

         Derived from Tables compiled by F. Fraser, Social Welfare Policy
         Secretariat, Canberra.

Australian Capital Territory, Tasmania and Western Australia (roughly 1:2,000 aged). Victoria and South Australia again have a much lower ratio while the Northern Territory has the lowest ratio of 1:850 aged. The financial allocations have minimal relationship to the ratio of centres to aged. The situation becomes more complicated when it is known that not all of the existing centres receive funds via the States Grants (Home Care) Act. In NSW for example, there are known to be approximately 515 centres, only 115 of which have received money under the States Grants Act. Also the two territories do not receive funds under the same agreements as the States but may receive funds either from separately appropriated Commonwealth Grants and/or locally raised funds such as the Community Development Fund in the Australian Capital Territory (Fraser, 1983).

Despite variations in funding the findings of the Extended Care Working Party of the Victorian Health Commission

(1981) on usage of centres, could well apply to senior citizen centres throughout Australia. This working party found that in Victoria there are 311 clubs (subsidised and unsubsidised) with total membership of 47,291 which represented 14.5% of the Victorian aged population. Attendance at the most important meeting each month corresponded to 5% of the total Victorian aged population and 36% of members. As only 5% of the aged attend the centres, the number of frail aged persons attending could be estimated to be considerably less than 5%. Therefore, although the intention was to provide a focal point for the provision of a wide range of social, recreational and welfare services for all aged persons within the community, in practice the centres cater for a small percentage of the population, are open for strictly limited periods and provide very litte apart from social events for the well aged (Victorian Health Commission, 1981).

As another attempt to meet the needs of aged Australians, the Commonwealth Government subsidises up to one-half of a salary for a welfare officer on a $1:$1 basis with State and/or local government contributions. The welfare officer must be employed in conjunction with a senior citizens' centre (irrespective of whether the centre is subsidised), and provide welfare services wholly or mainly for the aged. In 1980/81 $1.25 million was allocated under this program and since its inception in 1969 the Commonwealth has provided a total of $5.6 million for Welfare Officers for the aged.

Fifty-five welfare officers are currently being subsidised under the States Grants (Home Care) Act in NSW. Most of these are employed by local governments. However, a small number of voluntary, non-profit organisations also receive subsidies for welfare officers. In Victoria, 63 of the 212 Victorian municipalities employ welfare officers. To ensure that welfare officers provide services for which they are funded, the Commonwealth has suggested to the States the range of duties that a welfare officer should or could perform. The Commonwealth envisages the main function of a welfare officer is to ensure the development, co-ordination and continuing provision of the most appropriate welfare sources to meet the needs of the aged in the area. The services can be provided by a wide range of organisations. However, the development and co-ordination of such services is a major part of the welfare officer's duties. All States have acknowledged the guidelines but have not agreed to implement them.

The States Grants (Paramedical) Act (1969) is a companion to the previous Home Care Act. Indeed, both the States Grants (Home Care) Act (1969) and the States Grants (Paramedical Services) Act (1969) were enacted to correct the institutional approach to care, specifically to provide domiciliary services for those unable to afford private services. Under this legislation the Federal government makes grants on a dollar for dollar basis to the States for the provision of medical services wholly or mainly for the aged persons in their homes. The services that are usually provided are occupational therapy, speech therapy, chiropody and social work in conjunction with the above services.

The States have been slow to develop these services and even now only three States—South Australia, Victoria and Tasmania participate in this program. Not surprisingly, expenditure under this program has been nowhere near the magnitude of other Acts. Grants for paramedical services for 1982/83 are estimated to be $1.2 million (Australian Budget Statements, 1982).

DELIVERED MEALS

The Australian Government subsidises approved non-profit delivered meal services. The organisations providing these services typically include religious and charitable/benevolent agencies and local government bodies. These organisations can serve meals at senior citizens' centres but home help services and State Government instrumentalities are ineligible for subsidy. The Commonwealth Department of Social Security via its State branches administers this program. To date the only accountability 'meals on wheels' organisations have had is to provide quarterly returns, stating only numbers of meals served, upon which retrospective subsidies are calculated. The Department does not require financial statements from the services and does not implement policies on eligibility of clients, service procedures or charges for meals. The finance for the program comes from the National Welfare Fund (National Welfare Fund Act, 1969) and subsidies are allocated according to the formula set down in the Delivered Meals Subsidy Act. The subsidy now stands at 50¢ and 5¢ vitamin C supplement per meal. In 1981/82 a total of 9.6 million meals were served at a total cost of $4.2 million. Since its inception in 1969/70 the Commonwealth has provided a total of $22.8 million for service. In the latest Commonwealth budget, it was estimated that $5.6 million would be spent on this service during 1982/83. Table 6 sets out the details of funds, numbers of participating organisations and the year by year growth since 1969/70.

It can be seen from this Table that the numbers of organi-

TABLE 6:   DELIVERED MEALS - NUMBER OF MEALS, ORGANISATIONS
            AND EXPENDITURE, % GROWTH BY YEAR, 1969/70 TO 1981/82

Year	Funds		Organizations		Meals	
	$	% Change	Number	% Change	Number	% Change
1969/70	195,555	-	191	-	1,955,477	
1970/71	340,961	74	Not Available	-	Not Available	-
1971/72	337,582	-1	316	-	''	-
1972/73	586,777	74	348	10	3,864,474	-
1973/74	1,372,944	134	401	15	4,782,807	24
1974/75	1,490,292	9	450	12	5,334,363	12
1975/76	1,799,253	21	501	11	5,992,799	12
1976/77	1,911,173	6	560	12	6,601,658	10
1977/78	2,207,825	16	609	9	7,111,750	8
1978/79	2,279,981	3	633	4	7,651,874	8
1979/80	2,492,927	9	671	6	8,357,208	9
1980/81	3,623,797	45	714	6	8,947,352	7
1981/82	4,252,788	17	738	3	9,648,601	8
TOTAL	22,891,855				70,248,363	

Source: Annual Reports of Department of Social Security, 1969/70 to
          1981/82.
          Australian Budget Statements, 1982/83.

sations and meals over the twelve year period have more than tripled, while subsidies have increased eighteenfold. The largest percentage increases in funds correspond to adjustments made in the basic subsidy in the years 1973, 1974 and 1980. Changes in funding have not followed a smooth gradient by any means. In contrast to 'no-growth' in 1971/72, 1973/74 was a year of very marked increase (145%), an increment which was not sustained or repeated. Rather, there has been a pattern of a significant increase one year followed by a much smaller increment the following year. Upon closer study it can be seen that these increases do not correspond to increases in either the number of delivered-meals organisations or the number of meals provided.

In NSW, for the financial year 1981/82, nearly 3 million meals were served from 231 organisations, an 8% increase in the number of meals served from the previous year. Approximately 50% of those meals were served at senior citizen centres. As a ratio of the aged population, 4,004 meals were served per 1,000 of the population aged 60 plus, roughly .08% of a meal per aged person per week. Victoria provides roughly 35% of all meals produced yet even in this State the average is 103.6 meals per week per 1,000 elderly population or 0.1% of a meal per aged person per week. Differences in State participation under this program are presented in Table 7.

It can be seen that NSW and Victoria together receive roughly 66% of all funds provided per year. South Australia's involvement has decreased steadily since 1969/70, as has NSW, while the opposite has occurred in Victoria.

A Department of Social Security investigation into the services and organisations subsidised under this Act revealed two main types of organisations with different cost structures and operating methods. One type used hospital facilities to produce meals and were essentially transportation and serving agents. These organisations procured meals at a specified basic cost, delivered at cost price, utilised a proportion of the subsidy for running expenses and have surplus funds. They usually existed in rural sectors where community support was relatively abundant. Due to the cost savings associated with these factors, this group of organisations were financially sound and relatively satisfied with current subsidy and payment arrangements. The second group identified, prepared

TABLE 7:   DELIVERED MEALS SUBSIDY BY STATE,
AS PROPORTION OF TOTAL EXPENDITURE AND % YEARLY INCREASE, 1969/70 TO 1981/82*

Year	N.S.W. %	Victoria %	Queensland %	S.Aust. %	W.Aust. %	Tasmania %	Nth.Terr. %	A.C.T. %	Total $ 000s	% Change
1969/70	32	25	9	20	10	3	0	0.2	195.5	-
1970/71	37	32	7	13	9	2	.1	0.2	340.9	74
1971/72	35	30	8	14	8	3	.09	0.3	337.5	1
1972/73	33	32	9	13	8	4	.07	0.3	586.7	67
1973/74	33	32	9	12	9	4	.06	0.4	1,372.9	145
1974/75	32	32	10	12	10	4	.02	0.2	1,490.2	19
1975/76	32	33	11	11	10	4	.07	0.2	1,799.2	21
1976/77	31	28	11	14	11	4	0	0.5	1,911.1	6
1977/78	30	33	11	12	10	4	.1	0.4	2,207.8	16
1978/79	30	33	11	11	11	4	.1	0.5	2,279.9	3
1979/80	30	35	11	10	10	4	.1	0.5	2,492.9	9
1980/81	29	37	11	10	9	3	.1	0.5	3,626.8	45
1981/82	29	37	11	10	10	3	.2	0.4	4,252.8	17

* Totals may not add exactly due to rounding.

Source: Annual Reports of Department of Social Security, 1969/70 to 1981/82.

meals in the kitchens of senior citizen centres, town halls, councils, nursing homes or other facilities. Unlike the first group, these organisations had to purchase meal ingredients, provide kitchen staff and pay overheads. Not surprisingly, they were experiencing financial difficulties and were in need of increased subsidies.

The investigation also revealed considerable interstate differences. Victoria, as indicated earlier, has a greater input from local government authorities (70% of all councils) while NSW has a much lower local government component (5%). Further, there were considerable differences between administration by State offices of the Department of Social Security. For example, unlike Western Australia, 42% of NSW organisations had not been formally contacted since 1978. Meal production costs, vitamin C costs, meal charges and delivery costs were all found to vary markedly within and between States (Chartres, 1982). Examples of these State differences are that NSW hospitals provide (although now this has decreased) considerable support for meals on wheels services. Seventy percent of meals are provided by NSW hospitals whereas in Queensland it is the current policy of the Department of Health that meals cannot be provided from hospital kitchens. As a result, Queensland services have been establishing themselves as almost the sole users of Senior Citizen Centres' kitchens. Moreover, in Queensland, the decision of whether a client should continue receiving meals is primarily the task of the community nurse, while in NSW this can be done by a variety of people including the delivered meals co-ordinator (if one exists), the home care assessor or a local council community worker.

All States however, share the same dependence upon volunteer labour to deliver the meals and co-ordinate operations. As the subsidy relates only to meals, voluntary labour has been becoming increasingly difficult to procure as work and petrol costs have increased.

COMMUNITY HEALTH PROGRAM

The early 1970s saw the advent of the first Labor Government for some twenty odd years and a new emphasis upon community health. The Community Health Program (CHP) as it was known, marked formal governmental recognition of the dominance of curative, institutional interests in earlier health planning and budgeting. Although the CHP was never granted legislative status and never attained its objectives (partly because of fluctuating funding and commitment by the later Liberal Government from 1975), much of its resources went (and still do, though under State community services programs) to maintaining the chronically ill and disabled in their own homes and community.

At one stage, it was thought that this program would incorporate programs such as the home nursing subsidy. This did not eventuate however. Rather, successive decreases in Commonwealth funding produced progressive dismantling of the CHP. Now community health services are provided by each State Government. These services do not have a legislative base and statistics are not collected systematically in most States. NSW has just seen the placement of previously autonomous community health services under the auspices of the hospital sector.

Table 8 following sets out Commonwealth support for the Community Health Program between years 1973 and 1980, and also the funding provided by both Commonwealth and State governments. It is evident from these figures that in 1978 there was not only a significant drop in the percentage contribution of the Commonwealth, but also in the funding level. As a result, services and manpower were reduced (McKenzie, 1982). In 1981, the Commonwealth Government ceased to fund these community services under specific purpose grants, preferring instead to make an identifiable health grant within general revenue to the States. The funding in the identifiable grants was fixed at the 1980/81 rate plus an additional 10% for inflation for 1981/82. For 1982/83, the basic grant remained the same but with approximately a 21% addition. This alteration masked the devolution of Commonwealth responsibility for the program. As it coincided with the termination of cost-sharing agreements between the Commonwealth and State governments for acute hospital services, the community health program was forced to compete against the institutional sector for resources.

TABLE 8: COMMUNITY HEALTH PROGRAM - PROPORTIONAL CONTRIBUTION OF THE
COMMONWEALTH GOVERNMENT FOR CAPITAL AND OPERATING COSTS
AND FUNDING BY COMMONWEALTH AND STATE GOVERNMENTS, 1973 TO 1980

Year	% Commonwealth Support Capital Costs	Operating Costs	Commonwealth $000s*	State $000s*	Yearly Total $000s*
1973/74	100	100	12,840	0	12,840
1974/75	75	90	25,747	4,411	30,159
1975/76	75	90	47,139	8,310	55,449
1976/77	75	90	65,505	10,564	76,069
1977/78	50	75	66,038	28,907	94,945
1978/79	50	50	49,340	47,766	97,106
1979/80	50	50	54,180	51,549	105,730
1980/81	-	-	60,034	56,740	116,774
TOTAL			380,823	208,247	589,070

*   National projects which are 100% funded by Commonwealth, e.g.
Women's Refuges, have been excluded.

Source: Commonwealth Department of Health, Australia.

ASSISTANCE TO 'CARERS'

There is a growing literature on the needs and situation of carers—that is, people who look after somebody in their own home who could not otherwise manage by themselves. Much of this literature has pointed to the stress and demands experienced by these carers—the unshared responsibility, the lack of sleep and recreation, anxiety, family disruptions, financial burdens and ill-health (Hartshorn, 1953; Stevenson, 1976; Goldstein, Rognery and Wellin, 1981; Rowland, 1981; Gibson, 1980a, 1980b, 1982).

Australia has two benefits which provide some assistance and acknowledgement of the role of carers. The first, the Domiciliary Nursing Care Benefit (1972) is paid to an applicant for caring for a patient at home who would otherwise require institutional care. The patient must be over the age of sixteen and certified by a medical practitioner as requiring continuing care and by a registered nurse as receiving adequate nursing care. The second benefit, the Handicapped Children's Allowance (1975) is paid to a parent or guardian of a severely mentally or physically handicapped child who requires constant care and who is living in the family home. Allowances for substantially handicapped children were introduced in 1977. However, this latter amount depends on the parents' income and the additional costs incurred in caring for the child. At the end of the 1981 financial year, nearly 30,000 allowances were being paid, while total expenditure since 1975 has been $117.5 million.

Although both benefits were motivated (at least, in part) to ease the financial burden of caring for someone at home, the explicit intention of the Domiciliary Nursing Care Benefit (1972) was to encourage people to look after their aged relatives in their own home instead of having them admitted to nursing homes, hospitals or other institutions. This is reflected in the condition that each patient has to require such care at home that if she/he applied for admission to an approved nursing home, the application would be approved. Expenditure for this benefit in 1982/83 is estimated to be $22.6 million, $1.6 million higher than 1981/82 expenditure which is in response to the expected growth of 7% in the number of recipients (Australian Budget Papers, 1982/83). Table 9 sets out for the Domiciliary Nursing Care Benefit (DNCB) and Handicapped Children's Allowance (HAC) the number of beneficiaries within each State and total benefits, 1981/82.

NSW and the Australian Capital Territory combined have the highest number of beneficiaries (35%); Victoria (20%); Queensland (20%); South Australia and Northern Territory (9%); Western Australia (9%) and Tasmania (7%). The total figure of 18,153 beneficiaries, as an indicator of the number of carers or of severely ill or disabled people being cared for at home, is virtually useless due to the narrow eligibility, restrictive conditions and because it excludes those ill and disabled people who live alone. Many people are also unaware of the benefit's existance.

At the commencement of this article the disparity between funding for institutional and non-institutional services was mentioned. However, apart from the lack of funds directed to

TABLE 9:   DOMICILIARY NURSING CARE BENEFIT AND HANDICAPPED CHILDREN'S
            ALLOWANCE, EXPENDITURE AND RECIPIENTS BY STATES, 1981/82

State	Number of Beneficiaries		Benefits Paid $,000	
	D.N.C.B.	H.C.A.	D.N.C.B.	H.C.A.
New South Wales and Australian Capital Territory	6,321	9,111	7,176	7,559
Victoria	3,693	7,855	5,116	6,379
Queensland	3,659	3,771	3,985	3,127
South Australia and Northern Territory	1,607	2,907	1,760	2,492
Western Australia	1,658	2,542	1,769	2,054
Tasmania	1,215	859	1,365	689
TOTAL	18,153	27,045	21,172	22,300

Source: Annual Report of the Director General of Health, 1981/82.
         Annual Report of the Department of Social Security, 1981/82.

community and domiciliary services, the various programs
outlined above contain various shortcomings which seriously
impair their effectiveness. The Home Nursing Subsidy, for
example, relates only to the salaries of registered nurses.
Other costs such as transport and ancillary workers are not
provided. In addition the Act provides a different subsidy
according to whether the organisation was established before
or after the Act. Those organisations founded after 1956 can
only receive at maximum 50% of what pre-1956 organisations
receive per nursing position. However those nursing positions
which existed prior to 1956, a national total of 215 positions,
do not receive any support under this Act (or any other Act)
solely because they existed prior to the Act's introduction.
Despite these anomalies the Home Nursing Subsidy Act is
now being looked to by various State health authorities as a
means of augmenting funds. With the States Grants (Home
Care) Act, given the demonstrated poor utilisation of senior
citizens' centres relative to the inability of home help services
to provide adequate assistance, the continuing establishment

and support of these centres to the tune of 25% of State Grants (Home Care) expenditure appears inappropriate at the very least. It is also felt that the Delivered Meals legislation should be subsumed under the State Grants (Home Care) Act to improve its co-ordination and overlap with the above Act. There has been widespread dissatisfaction with the Domiciliary Nursing Care Benefit and its application on the grounds that the requirement to have a nurse call every two weeks to check the patient's care is wasteful in times of high demand upon home nursing services; that the benefit is too low; that it has not kept pace with increases in the cost of living and that the provision for the carer to be absent from the patient for only short absences for shopping or business matters is unrealistic and without compassion. Moreover, the benefit discriminates against those who live alone.

However not all of the difficulties facing community and domiciliary support services are directly attributable to legislative problems or lack of government support. The awareness of these services is low. Most of the recent Australian research upon knowledge of community and domiciliary services has studied the knowledge of the frail or disabled elderly. One study surveyed 501 people aged 60 years and over in Sydney, Australia's largest city. Just over half the sample (57%) indicated that they were aware of any services for older people needing help at home. Of this 57%, 27% could specify one service, a further 21% two services, and only 3% three or more. The remaining 6% gave only general or vague responses. Of those services mentioned, meals on wheels was the most commonly known (43% of respondents). Domiciliary nursing and home help were known to 21% and 13% respectively. Other types of domiciliary care were virtually or totally unknown (Gibson, 1982). Another smaller random survey of older residents within a local government area revealed that few of the elderly residents used community and domiciliary services even though they indicated that they had problems with transport, shopping and health needs. Furthermore, 22% of this sample (250 respondents) thought that they would probably go into an old persons' home as an answer to these unmet needs (Douglas and Eyland, 1982). Knowledge of services is an important determinant of their use and, although both studies are based upon small sample sizes, they do yield disturbing implications for home support services.

Part of the ability of the community and domiciliary services to maintain and preferably increase the quality of life and options open to recipients requires not only referral to such services by hospitals and nursing homes but also within the range of services labelled 'community and domiciliary care'. Unfortunately referral between services does not occur as frequently as would be expected. A study of referral to Home Care branches in NSW revealed that only 18% of the 50 branches surveyed said that meals on wheels organisations frequently referred clients to them and 75% indicated that such referrals happened "occasionally" (Keens and Graycar, 1983). Consequently it is rare for an ill or disabled person to be receiving more than one domiciliary service (Philips, 1981).

The predominance of a curative, medical and institutional approach has resulted in a paucity of data and of literature relating to the activities and processes of home support services. Consequently, it is impossible to gain a reliable figure illustrating the country's usage of home support services. As it was mentioned earlier, the last national Census on the characteristics of home nursing patients was collected in 1974. Since this time the only national information collected for home nursing pertains solely to crude measures such as the total number of patients visited, kilometres travelled, number of nurses employed and funding provided under the Home Nursing Act. Details as to the average length of visits, frequency of visits, turnover rate, referral sources and patient profiles can only be obtained from individual agencies and then with differential success. Similarly, with the delivered meals subsidy. Even less national information is available on the utilisation of services provided under the States Grants, Home Care and Paramedical Services Acts. Even rough estimates are not possible as some States (Queensland and South Australia) cannot even provide figures on clients or numbers. Fortunately, each State has begun to investigate ways of establishing community and domiciliary data bases.

It is possible to derive some idea of the need for home support services via the Australian Bureau of Statistics Survey of Handicapped Persons (1981) which estimated that 83% of those who are moderately and severely disabled in the areas of self care and mobility (973,400 persons) live outside of institutions. The survey revealed only 25% of all handicapped received any non-medical assistance at home. The majority (57%) received only one type of assistance and, of these, 48% were severely handicapped. Although the number of services received increased with age and severity of handicap, only 40% of people who had moderate or severe handicaps received two services. Irrespective of degree of handicap or number of services received, nearly 60% of those who received assistance with meals, gained it four or more times a week. In contrast, assistance with domestic work was only received four times weekly by 8%. The majority (50%) gained help once a week. Thus it can be seen that few handicapped persons receive many, if any, domiciliary services. A failure which the survey revealed had forced many handicapped persons into institutions.

At present by far the most frequent form of care provided is informal care, that is, care given by friends, neighbours and relatives (Howe, 1979). However, demographic trends in combination with social changes are altering the capacity of the family, and particularly of females, to provide voluntary support. One of these factors is the change in the over 65 years population which indicates that the proportion of 'old-old' people will increase by 33%. Other factors are decreases in family size, reducing the availability of potential family support; fewer 'never-married' women in Australia than ever before (for every 100 elderly persons in 1901 there were 8.7 unmarried women aged 45 to 59; today there are 4.1); increasing female participation in the labour force (an increase over the past decade from 30% to 45%) and, internal migration within Australia from the colder southern States to warmer northern States which has placed geographical constraints upon the ability of the family to care. Thus the chronically ill and disabled may have to rely more on formal programs for needed support. Similar trends have been pointed out in America by Reif and Estes (1982).

Table 10 sets out the projections for the composition of Australia's aged population. Although the projected numerical increase of the population aged over 60 (females) and 65 (males) shall be only one million by the year 2000, it is the percentage increase within each age bracket that is causing concern to health and welfare economists, administrators and providers. The numbers of elderly under 75, as a proportion

TABLE 10:   PROJECTIONS OF THE COMPOSITION
                   OF THE AUSTRALIAN AGED POPULATION

Age	1980 No.	2000 No.	Increase %
Under 75*	1,200,000	1,565,000	+ 30.4
75 to 84	400,000	715,000	+ 78.7
85 and over	94,000	220,000	+134.0
TOTAL	1,694,000	2,500,000	+ 47.5

*   Females aged 60 and males aged 65.

Source: Australian Bureau of Statistics, Series D Population Projection.

of the total aged shall fall from 71% (1980) to 63% in 2000 (projected). However, those aged between 75 and 84 as a proportion of the total aged shall increase to 29% by the year 2000. Similarly, those aged over 85 shall comprise 9% of the total aged. Thus, that portion of the elderly population which is the greatest consumer of health and welfare services shall show the greatest increase. Awareness of these population trends and the expense of institutional care has produced considerable interest in home support services as a mechanism for containing the cost of aged health and welfare. Concomitantly, with the increasing emphasis upon reduction of health care expenditure, greater demand shall be directed to community and domiciliary services, services which are struggling to meet existing demand.

The various Commonwealth Acts and programs which constitute community and domiciliary services in Australia have been repeatedly criticised for their unco-ordinated administration, inadequate coverage and poor funding. However, the greatest failure of all the legislation described above is its failure to provide home support services with an identity and status which is consistent with their inherent and potential value. Obviously it was cheaper to rely upon volunteers and to fund only certain aspects of a needed service—for example, the cost of a meal, than comprehensively address and fund all aspects of the program. Australia is presently trying to rectify the consequences of this ad hoc and fragmented response which has

resulted from the predominance of the vested interests of curative, medical and institutional sectors. Seven reports have recommended improvements in the present system of service provision. A further report has been added recently to this dusty
pile. The latest report comes from the Macleay Committee, an
expenditure inquiry into the funding and administration of accommodation and home support services for the aged. This
report essentially proposes a reduction in the number of programs; responsibility for all aged programs to be brought under
the Minister for Health, modifications to financial arrangements to remove disincentives for the expansion of home care
services, greater control over the numbers and use of nursing
home beds, the provision of care in hostels by domiciliary services and, more broadly, the reallocation of savings from the
institutional sector to community care. The focus of the report
is to rationalise the administrative divisions and complexities
underlying the provision of Commonwealth funds by transferring to the Commonwealth Department of Health the responsibility for all home support programs and devolve over five
years, responsibility to the States by making payments to aged
services via general tax-sharing agreements. The former re-
structuring assumes that one departmental umbrella will pave
the way for rational, effective and responsible provision of
services, while the latter abrogates any responsibility for involvement in aged care beyond determining how much the
Federal Government is prepared to contribute.

This report has formed the basis of the national frail aged
health policy of the recently elected Australian Labor Party.
The new government has rejected the report's recommendation to return all responsibility to the States for the provision
of programs through tax-sharing agreements in favour of 90%
Commonwealth and 10% State funding across all programs
including institutional services. While the States acknowledge
that this removes the anomalies and disincentives that presently exist, there is great reluctance to enter into an agreement whereby the Commonwealth can slowly withdraw their
support leaving the States with not only the administration
but also the financial burden of providing services. To rectify
the existing imbalance between institutional and non-institutional services, the new Minister for Health has said for a
period of three years, the financial allocation made for the

services described above shall be supplemented by an additional $35 million per year. To produce by 1986/87 an annual increment of $105 million. A separate $15 million has been promised for community health services. Legislative gaps and program anomalies are planned to be removed by replacing existing legislation by three main programs: Community Care; Residential and Nursing Home Care. All programs to be administered by the Commonwealth Department of Health. Unlike the previous Federal Government, the Labor Government sees a broader role for the Commonwealth Government. The possibility of national minimum standards is being considered.

The return to power of a Labor Government has injected optimism into the health and welfare sectors depleted by the gap between the transfer of public responsibilities onto private individuals and the ability of individuals and families to care for family members. However, a number of elements of the new Government's 'Frail Aged Policy' are causing concern for providers of home support services. The dominant concern is that the $35 million supplement for these services is insufficient on a national basis, particularly for all the programs which urgently require funds. There is considerable concern too that the frequent prescription of regional assessment teams as a solution to inappropriate admission to nursing homes is not seen to depend upon the availability of community and domiciliary services. Furthermore, the aim that the assessment teams determine access to non-institutional services, particularly welfare services according to the 'health needs' of the clients, is seen as ignoring the significance of social and familial factors. The over-riding implication being to place the responsibility for all needs of the aged, social and health needs, within a health model. As it has been extensively pointed out, not all the aged are sick and not all require health services. Thus the proposal that access to domiciliary services be determined by an assessment team according to 'health needs' introduces the danger that health care solutions shall be applied to non-health care needs. Moreover, the emphasis on assessment teams is felt to be strongly upon their gatekeeping function—an effective way of containing or reducing the consumption of expensive services by elderly people.

The Australian Labor Party has also expressed its intention to ultimately allocate the money to the States for institutional and non-institutional services in undifferentiated block grants (Blewitt, 1983). For those involved in the provision of services for the frail aged, particularly of home support services, such arrangements cause concern given the power of institutional and medical services and the recent experience of community health since the conclusion of specific purpose grants.

Attempts to rectify existing legislation and administrative structures need to be made with due respect to compromises that have been reached with existing arrangements and within and between States for example, it is a popular idea to make local government responsible for the co-ordination and even provision of many services. Such strategies rely upon the involvement and expertise of local government. In Victoria programs requiring considerable local council input would have a greater degree of success given that State's longer history of local government involvement in health and welfare services. In NSW however, the same strategy would run into immediate difficulties. In addition, the sudden concern at the aging of Australia's population and the cost of health and welfare carries the danger that home support services shall be seen only from the perspective of the needs of the elderly rather than increasing the ability of such services to cater for all sections of society who also require assistance at home. Much of Australia's provision of community and domiciliary services is directed towards the older age groups even though the number of children placed in residential care is increasing continually, even though there are more single parents than ever before and despite the needs of the increasing number of disabled. The greatest need of home support services in Australia is money, money, money. The initiatives taken by the new Federal Government will be watched closely by many to see if the rhetoric shall be matched by action.

REFERENCES

Australian Budget Papers, "Budget Statements, 1982–83", 1982/83 Budget Paper No. 1, Australian Government Publishing Service, Canberra, Australia, 1982.
Australian Budget Papers, "Payment To and For the States, the Northern Territory and Local Government Authorities, 1982–83,", 1982/83 Budget Paper No. 7, Australian Government Publishing Service, Canberra, Australia, 1982.

Australian Bureau of Statistics, "Handicapped Persons Australia 1981", Catalogue No. 4343.0, Australian Bureau of Statistics, Canberra, Australia, 1982.

Australian Labor Party, Health Workshop, "The Frail Aged", February 4/5th, 1983.

Chartres, N., "Delivered Meals Subsidy Act: Investigation into Services Provided by Organisations and Subsidies Under the Act", Department of Social Security, Western Australia, Subsidies Section, 1982.

Coombs, E.M., "Year to Date Comparison with Previous Financial Year: The State of the Home Care Service of New South Wales". Report to the State Executive Committee, Home Care Service of New South Wales, Sydney, Australia. Unpublished. February, 1983.

Douglas, V. and Eyland, F., "Usage of Community Services in the Hunter's Hill Local Government Area", Hunter's Hill Municipal Council, Sydney, Australia, 1982.

Fraser, F., "Data Base for Commonwealth Assisted Accommodation and Home Support Services—Aged and Disabled", Social Welfare Policy Secretariat, Canberra, Australia, 1983.

Gibson, D.M., "Knowledge of Community Services Amongst the Aged". Working Paper No. 31, Ageing and the Family Project, Research School of Social Sciences, Australian National University, Canberra, Australia, 1982.

Gibson, M.J., "An International Update on Family Care for the Ill Elderly", *Ageing International*, Vol. 9, No. 1, Spring 1982, pp. 11–14.

Gibson, M.J., "Family Support for the Elderly in International Perspective: Part I", *Ageing International*, Vol. 7, No. 2, Summer 1980a, pp. 12–16.

Gibson, M.J., "Family Support for the Elderly in International Perspective: Part II, Policies and Programs", *Ageing International*, Vol. 7, No. 4, Winter 1980b, pp. 13–19.

Goldstein, V., Regnery, G. and Wellin, E., "Caretaker Role Fatigue", *Nursing Outlook*, Vol. 29, No. 1, January 1981, pp. 24–30.

Hartshorn, A.E., "The Social Implications of Ill Health as they Affect the Family". Proceedings of the Fourth National Conference of Social Work, Australia, 1953, p.36.

Henderson, R.F. and Lewis, R.B., "Local Government and Personal and Community Services" in R.B. Scotton and H. Ferber (eds.), *Public Expenditures and Social Policy in Australia*, Volume II, The First Fraser Years, 1976–78, Longman Cheshire, Melbourne, Australia, 1980.

Howe, A., "Family Support of the Aged", *Australian Journal of Social Issues*, Vol. 14, No. 4, November 1979.

Keens, C. and Graycar, A., "Home Help Services in Australia", Social Welfare Research Centre, University of New South Wales, Sydney, Australia, 1983, in press.

The Honourable Leo Macleay. Speech to the Australian House of Representatives on the Report of the Standing Committee on Expenditure, 28th October 1982, Hansard, pp. 27, 32–2735, 1982.

McKenzie, R., "The State of the Australian Health Care System: Crisis for Community". Paper presented at Royal Australian Nursing Federation, Standards for Nursing Practice, National Conference, Melbourne, Australia, 13–15th October 1982.

Philips, T.J., "A Comparative Cost Evaluation of Alternative Modes of Long-term Care for the Aged", Part II: Final Technical Report, School of Health Administration, University of New South Wales, July 1981.

Queensland Department of Health, Advisory Committee on the Care of the Aged, "First Consolidated Report", Queensland, Australia, 1981.

Reif, L. and Estes, C.L., "Long-term Care: New Opportunities for Professional Nursing" in *Nursing in the 1980s: Crises, Opportunities, Challenges*, L.M. Aiken (ed.), Philadelphia, Pennsylvania, U.S.A., J.B. Lippincott, 1982, pp. 147–181.

Rowland, D.T., "Sixty-five Not Out: Consequences of the Ageing of Australian Population", Institute of Public Affairs (NSW), Australia, 1981.
Stevenson, C., "Dedication—A Report of a Survey on Caring for the Aged at Home", Council of the Ageing, Sydney, Australia, 1976.
Victorian Health Commission, Working Party on extended care of aged or disabled persons. Discussion Document, Victoria, Australia, 1981.

Report of a Mission from France to Review Care Provided to the Aged in Sweden

Patrick Terroir

A GENERAL QUESTION

For some years the countries of the occidental world have been confronted with the growth of a very aged population and the difficulties involved in assuring that population the medical and social care which it requires to preserve an independent place in society.

For the first time a significant proportion of the population is made up of people over the age of sixty-five and the same questions are emerging everywhere.

The appearance of a certain number of pathological conditions which are found more frequently in aging, the processes of aging organisms, call for the development of special kinds of care.

Along with active care directed to restoration and cure over limited periods of time there is a need for medical supervision in which regularity is more important than intensity, as well as a need for services which are effective in supporting the ability to carry out the activities of daily living. These services and this help must often be provided to older people over long periods of time while their status is practically stabilized and must sometimes be provided throughout the last years of life.

It is considered that the organisation of care which is re-

This study tour occurred on September 9–19, 1980. At the time of this study, Patrick Terroir was Chief of the Bureau P.1. Social Security Administration, Ministry of Health and of Social Security. This report was published in *Années,* the journal of the Center for Liaison, Study, Information and Research on the Problems of Older People (CLEIRPPA) No. 104. March, 1981 Paris, France. The translation is by Brahna Trager.

Requests for reprints can be sent to the author at: 68 Avenue de Saxe, Paris 75015, France.

sponsive to these needs is absolutely fundamental to the lives of these people as well as to society.

In recent years France has implemented four important activities on behalf of its older population:

—The elimination of hospices (old people's homes) in which conditions were especially deficient.
—The development of home care. But home nursing is still limited compared to home help services, and more generally compared with services which are social in nature.
—The introduction of treatment personnel in retirement homes (medical treatment sections) in order to enable older people to continue to live in them if they require care.
—Creation of long-stay hospitals to make sure that those who are the most seriously ill and the most dependent will be accepted. It is in this sector that the largest number of beds has been created. In all of these situations the cost of housing is the responsibility of the individual, who can have recourse to social assistance. Treatment is covered by medical insurance. (Social Security covers everyone in France.) The main thrust of public policy at the present time is along the lines of developing home care services and the "medicalization" of retirement homes. It was therefore the two following themes that the mission planned to analyze in Sweden:
—How should the division between home care and institutional care be achieved?
—Within the institutional system, which is preferable, a method which is more like hospitalization or a "medicalized" social service structure?

THE PROGRAM

In addition to the focus of the study it is possible in such a mission to discover two kinds of general lessons. The first arises from a situation in which one finds oneself alone, confronting one's subject—a situation which a civil servant in the administration, and, I imagine, the majority of those who work in such enterprises or organizations rarely meets. The second is that one never has the opportunity to undertake in-depth studies of this kind in order to develop a dossier in one's own country—at least in my administrative experience.

The program outlined by the Swedish Institute included meetings with directors of the central administration: The National Agency for Health and Welfare, the Center for Studies and Planning of local collectives (SPRI), of the local administration: the Bureau of social assistance for Jonköping, an association of older people and an institute for research in Gerontology (located in Jonköping).

Additionally there were a number of visits in Stockholm as well as in the provinces to establishments for social care: retirement homes, congregate living facilities, residential hotels; to service centers for home helps (the "samaritaines"), as well as to medical establishments: Long-stay hospitals, nursing homes and home care services.

The only gap in this rich and varied circuit, which I was unable to fill, was that I was unable to meet with central organizations having the responsibility for definition and development of a national policy for the care of the aged. But decentralized Sweden has no parallel to our Parisian administration in which uniform directives are developed and which, in large part, carries responsibility for resources, for their financing or for the regulations by which they function.

I was aware, of course, that I was shown the best and the most successful examples, and I also understood that I would be unable to extract a general picture of services in Sweden, a country in which local powers have developed such competence. But I was looking for lessons and it was as well to find them in their most advanced versions. As for the more profound problems, they are obviously the same everywhere.

IF FRANCE WERE SWEDEN

Table 1 below presents a comparison in which the last column describes the resources which would be available in France if the same density prevailed as they do at present in Sweden. This table, in which it is appropriate to take the numbers in the order of magnitude because of the habitual heterogeneity of statistical categories, permits us to outline

TABLE 1

The table below presents a comparison in which the resources which France would have appear in the last column if similar density (to those in Sweden) are applied.

	Sweden	France	If France were Sweden there would be*
Total Population	8,314,000	53,373,000	
65 years +	1,300,000	7,300,000	8,300,000
80 years +	266,000	1,500,000	1,700,000
National Health Expenditures[1]	31.4 billion	151 billion	202 billion
Health Care personnel			
Physicians	13,000	91,500	83,600
Nurses	21,916	152,500	140,262
Number of medical consultations (per year)	18,000	168,000	116,000
Hospitals			
Acute care (Beds)	43,000	360,000	
Psychiatric (Beds)	30,000	139,000	
	73,000	500,000	467,000
intermediate		68,000	258,000
long stay	46,000	50,000	
Total	119,000	618,000	725,000
Housing for the aged			
retirement homes	60,600	300,000	
Congregate Housing Service flats	28,000	90,000	
	88,600	390,000	500,000
Home helps (for the aged)			
Personnel	73,400	60,000	411,040
Persons assisted	340,000	340,000	1,904,000

*This column is obtained by applying the same density of resources which exists in proportion to the population of Sweden to the population of France. The multiplicative coefficients used are 6.4 when the resources are intended for the entire population: they are 5.6 when they are intended principally for the aged.
[1]In Francs

some of the characteristics of Sweden as compared with France: the population is older, the resources for care in the city are not as great, hospital beds are slightly less numerous for short-term care but much more numerous for intermediate and long-term care, the system of social housing is more developed.

Sweden thus presents a high ratio of social housing and hospitals for the older population, at the same time that it has established very important means for home care (of the number of home helps). The medical sector and the social sector thus appear to have developed at the same rhythm but in a separate manner.

I. A Too Precise Separation Between Social Care and Health Care

Sweden, like France, and doubtless many other countries as well, distinguishes two spheres of intervention and competence, each of which is distinctly separated: the social domaine which combines services which assist with social functioning when this capacity is difficult or absent (retardation in children, functionally limited or handicapped people, the aged), and the health sphere which administers and organizes medical and hospital systems.

Dependent older persons are placed "at the crossroads." Because of their handicap or illness they require medical and paramedical care, but their need is principally for nursing care which is neither a need for specialized technology nor active medical intervention. They have an equal need for social assistance with activities of daily living: household maintenance and cooking. Above all, during the last years of life they have a right to a live in society which provides as much warmth as possible.

A. The Development of Social Care

A very large number of extremely important services have been developed in Sweden which permit older persons to live out a pleasant old age. On the day of retirement the retiree usually receives a visit from a social worker who estimates what his needs for help may be, if adaptation of housing is necessary, and informs him about the equipment and services which the commune and the county can make available.

1. The "Samaritaines" (Home Helps). At the initiative of local authorities and thanks to the support of the state which provides a subvention of 35% of the costs of these services, numerous home helps make it possible for a large number of older persons, who are incapable of managing activities of daily living alone, to remain in their own homes.

Because of their organization their administration is much simpler in Sweden than it is in France since they are entirely dependent on the municipality. The cost of the service to the participant is the responsibility of the community and is related to its income. The French system, on the other hand, includes a multiplicity of services and a great diversity in the costs of providing care.

This kind of help in Sweden has recently been improved in two directions:

— In order to insure a better team spirit and to extract useful information from their experience, the Samaritaines meet at the beginning of each day to report on the preceding day and to discuss the tasks for the day. More broadly the policy is to increase the status of the home help and to enrich their work experience in order to attract younger workers who are better trained and more stable.

— In several cities night patrols have been formed, charged with the responsibility for the safety of older persons and performing essential services needed by those who are most dependent: turning them in bed; managing incontinence.

— Finally it is indicated that the municipality of Stockholm has decided to eliminate all of the heavy detail involved in calculations related to the resources of participants and to provide those who need them with the services of home helps without charge.

Difficulties involved in the provision of these services are not new: personnel turnover, the frequently encountered problem of reducing the amount of help provided to an individual recipient of service.

When the family assumes responsibility for the functions

which would require the services of a home help it is entitled to receive the equivalent of the salary of that personnel.

2. Among the very numerous kinds of equipment and social services developed on behalf of older people, special notice should be taken of:

—A very advanced method for the assumption of responsibility for the costs of transportation. All older people are entitled to a book of tickets which allows them to have a certain number of taxi rides at a very reduced rate each month. Those with health problems never pay the costs of necessary transportation to hospitals or health centers.
—There are a very large number of meals centers. Older people may also lunch in the schools for a modest price.
—A large number of activities centers open to all of the inhabitants of the neighborhood have been established.
—Buses for heavy cleaning services circulate regularly.
—People can request that the postman, instead of simply delivering the mail, knock at the door to verify that everything is going well.

As in France the use of the retirement home has been abandoned in favor of arrangements more closely resembling individual housing.

Translated into our administrative language these structures have for several years been oriented toward congregate housing or boarding homes (in Sweden they are called residential hotels or service flats) with several groups of about ten apartments in one or two buildings around a unit of services and supervision.

These apartments are very modern with two or three rooms, and are equipped with those fixtures which are best adapted to the needs of the aging: ample clearance, accessible bathrooms, adjustable sinks, cookers equipped with safety devices (they are, incidentally, the same type of apartments which are found in special housing for the handicapped).

Services which are traditional for this type of establishment are provided: rehabilitation, occupational activities, crafts, looms for weaving, ceramics, carpentry shops, leisure activities and entertainments, gymnastics and physical therapy.

The highly perfected system of alarms is an obvious source

of pride in these establishments: along with buttons relayed to a luminous central console a "passive alert" system signals when an individual has not used the bathroom by a certain time in the morning.

There is, of course, a long waiting list for this type of apartment. It is composed of people who are either unable to remain in present housing because it is too old or is poorly situated, or because safety requirements or isolation make a change necessary.

Additional funding is planned to help with modernization or adaptation of old housing.

At times questions arise as to whether these apartments may not be a bit too "grand": the kitchens which are so sophisticated may not be used frequently by the inhabitant or by the home help; the workshops may sometimes be left empty by the pensioners. Nevertheless, enquiries and studies which have been conducted indicate that people do want this kind of arrangement.

One must also emphasize the very remarkable experiments with integration in housing for older people in central areas of housing and services for other sections of the population. At Hogsatra near Stockholm the same buildings are used by children, adults and the aged, and the results indicate that it is not simply a theoretical integration.

3. The system of allowances guarantees autonomy and freedom of choice. It is useful to emphasize the fact that old people can live alone only if they have adequate resources, and that numerous admissions to institutions often have their origin in inadequate income.

Sweden has established a pension system in two stages: a base sum is available to everyone without reference to resources. Beyond that, an amount is calculated on the basis of previous employment or professional income.

Above all, there exists a certain equality in the cost concerning the different means of housing. The commune is responsible, acording to the resources of the individual, for a portion of the costs of housing, whether the person lives in his own home or in an institution. For people who have only the basic allotment this becomes the total responsibility in either case. The only exception is that regulations concerning retirement homes have not yet advanced: the pension is given to the institution which only provides a certain amount of pocket money to the individual. Apparently a law is being drafted which will do away with this distinction.

As has been indicated above, responsibility for the costs of the home help is dependent upon personal resources.

Within the social sector one may conclude that the maintenance of the individual in his own home is the preferred method; in any case there is no economic incentive to enter an institution as may be the case in France where assistance with the cost of housing is limited to the housing allotment which is rather low. It should be emphasized, however, that supplementary services have been established—meals, transportation, leisure time activities.

B. But Social Services Stop at the Frontiers of the World of Health Care

Aging affects the functional status of the individual and this is frequently exacerbated by related illnesses. Social intervention then becomes insufficient: the need (except in acute phases) then is for nursing and paramedical care.

If these services cannot be brought to the place where the person lives—whether it is his own home, a retirement home, a boarding home, it becomes inevitable that the individual be uprooted and admitted to a medical institution. For reasons which were initially institutional Sweden finds itself in this situation:

1. Institutional logic. Sweden is a very decentralized country in which local authorities have full control of the resources entrusted to them.

—Social policy in favor of the aged (provision of home helps, special housing) is within the jurisdiction of the communes which balance their expenditures against community tax revenues.
—Health policy (institutions and personnel) is the responsibility of the "counties" (the equivalent of our departments or regions in France) which also levy a special tax.
—In this area the role of the central state is only to develop legislative reform, to offer good counsel or incentives and, of course, to provide general regulations.

Thus, each level has full control of the policy which it expects to implement with equal emphasis on political legitimacy and financial resources. Because spheres of control are precisely defined there is, of course, no need for arbitration.

Dependent old people find themselves on the borders of these respective spheres because their need is for care which is "medico-social."

The fact is that maintenance of older people at home encounters multiple difficulties with respect to "medicalization". If, as we have seen, a large number of home helps are serving dependent old people, it is not possible for the communes to employ nurses and health aides to provide the needed paramedical care since this personnel is answerable to the county.

On the other hand the counties are limited in their ability to provide service: care in the city remains primarily the responsibility of physicians and nurses of the district who do not have enough service available and whose functions do not include responsibility to assure care to these people.

Therefore, older people, when they need paramedical services, have to go to day hospitals regularly, and when they are no longer able to go they must be admitted to a long-stay hospital. On the other hand, a return to their own homes after a hospital stay is difficult because continuity of medical supervision and supportive maintenance is not possible.

Nevertheless, in practice, certain nuances should be included in this general view:

— Home helps provide paramedical care in certain cases. In fact people with massive handicaps are able to have five to six hours of home help service daily and then their services go beyond simple household tasks. In these situations a part of the cost is reimbursed by the county to the commune on a case-by-case basis for the hours employed in these services.
— Certain communes, of which Stockholm is one, have established night patrols which provide 'de facto" paramedical care.
— Confronted by the growth of hospitalization and the difficulties related to the discharge of the patients who no longer need active medical care, a certain number of

hospitals have established home care services using hospital personnel.

The same is true in boarding homes and retirement homes for the aged. It is difficult for the communes to employ paramedical personnel, and consequently to keep people who become ill or handicapped. It appears that several years ago retirement homes employed paramedical personnel and were able to assure essential services. This medicalization appeared to be insufficient and the combination of the healthy with invalids was considered shocking. As a result when an individual who lives in a retirement home or residential hotel requires treatment a transfer is made to a hospital. One director of a residence for older people described her situation as functioning well because the physician who came there on a freelance basis worked at the hospital and she therefore had an entree.

Nevertheless the retirement homes which have maintained the oldest residents, because of the period in which they were established, have been obliged to have recourse to nurses and nurses' aides because placements in long-term care centers are not available.

The counties therefore accept the responsibility for expenses related to such care but the communes would like to see the counties accept full responsibility for these establishments which they consider do not belong within their jurisdiction.

Paradoxically it is in one of the rare private retirement homes established by the middle class population of Stockholm that the equivalent of our medical treatment sections was installed. This home holds to the policy of allowing their pensioners to remain as long as they do not require intensive medical treatment. It has therefore added a team of nurses and nurses' aides (a total of ten) which is able to provide care to twenty-two of the ninety pensioners who are housed there.

2. A Response Which Is Necessarily Hospitalization. In the absence of care adapted to the need of the aged people who are limited in the capacity to undertake activities of daily living in their usual environment, there is no way to avoid shifting old people into the hospital from the moment they require the simplest medical measures.

—The result of this, first, congestion in medical services because of aged people who are admitted although in most instances hospitalization is medically useless, and who remain for long periods in the absence of adequate services of following up and measures which ensure continuity of care. Thus, in spite of their relatively large number, hospitals for long and intermediate stay are unable to accept all of the people who require a medical or paramedical environment.

—The general response to the need for care which old people and certain of the handicapped have, is service in long-stay hospitals.

It appears that two types of service for long-stay care exist in Sweden. The first is usually like a general hospital, or what we would call a center for intermediate and long stay. The objectives of these centers are to provide care, treatment and rehabilitation in order that the individual may return to an autonomous existence either at home or in an institution. Following this treatment and rehabilitation, a portion of these people remain for a long period or for the remainder of their lives.

Local facilities for long stay which are generally smaller in size provide a secondary recovery or transitional phase of care. People either come directly from the care of the physician when treatment or rehabilitation are useless, or from intermediate care centers when their pathological problems have been stabilized.

In both cases, however, this is a type of hospital institution for medical care and paramedical support. These establishments do not accept healthy people even if they are the husbands or wives of the hospitalized persons and the atmosphere, like the personnel, is rigidly that of a hospital—impersonal rooms with one or several beds, wide corridors, white coats. Efforts have been made, however, to bring some life into these establishments: activities such as weaving, carpentry, gymnastics have been made available to pensioners who generally use them very little, either because their condition makes it impossible or because the personnel have been unable to find a way to interest them. Some long-stay services have more success in this than others, and in one which is near Stockholm at Lidingo, very modern in style, closer in architecture to a "rest home," the people are involved in numerous activities, even printing a journal and considering themselves too busy to participate in physical therapy.

Nevertheless, in all these services, justification for a hospital environment is hardly apparent: the people housed in them are almost never in need of a level of medical care such as would be provided in a hospital. On the contrary, one is inclined to think that the hospital environment is more inconvenient than useful when it is a matter of spending the last years of one's life there.

The physicians who were questioned admitted that close to 80% of the people who are in long-stay services should be someplace else, either in their own homes or in social institutions. But in that case it would be impossible to provide some of the needed treatment. In the absence of a more suitable type of care, recourse to hospital-like establishments remains the only response to the needs of the aged, and this results in the rejection of a population of older people with functional limitations and the need to organize their transfer when they become ill or handicapped by physical changes. Finally the analysis of the pathology of aging has not really succeeded in demonstrating its singularity and the confusion between aging and illness has developed rapidly.

On the economic and financial side one should add that no financial participation by the individual is required in long-stay services during the first year, and after that, a contributions of 30 francs a day ($6 at the time of the report) is asked. Therefore, in practically all cases the long-stay choice is more advantageous than a retirement home or a boarding home and even the expenses of a normal household.

According to the information provided, the daily cost in the intermediate and long-stay hospital is about 400 francs a day.

The ratio of personnel to patient is greater than that provided in France (0.6 to 0.7 for medical personnel compared with 0.4 in France).

In order to avoid the hazards of hospitalization several hospitals have established home care services. Their introduction by social workers in such hospitals as the one at Rosalund in Stockholm, or by chiefs of medicine at Motala or Kalmar, have enabled these services to attempt to discharge older people from the hospital systematically. The pattern of these services is one which includes nurses, nurses' aides and physical therapists. They call upon home helps and work with the family with whom the return home is decided in the course of a long interview with the chief of medicine.

Such services have made it possible to return people to their homes even if they require concentrated care and are isolated. The night patrol makes regular visits and may be called upon in emergencies. It ensures patient safety, maintenance of treatment regimes and therapeutic movement for bedfast patients. The physician who is responsible for home care has funds available for the adaptation of housing which may be seriously deficient in facilities for care of the severely limited patient. In order to secure return home more easily the services always assure the individual that return to the long-stay center will be arranged immediately if either the individual or the family desire it. Some families, therefore, readily accept responsibility for the care of a sick or handicapped grandparent for a number of months each year. These services are also used in situations of terminal illness.

At Motala the home care services provide care for about 50 people a day, the majority with cardiovascular disease, cancer, neurological problems or dermatitis. About 40% of the sick in 1979 lived alone. The care provided was primarily nursing care: treatment of ulcers, or pain, placement of catheters and catheter care, monitoring of blood pressure, infusion. The daily cost was upward of 168 frances ($35) in 1979 (as against 550 francs in an intermediate or long-stay center).

These services are still very limited in number and remain in the experimental stage. The single real difference with France is found in the level of the discussion, for in practice we have very little home care service available.

On the whole, older people are hospitalized more frequently in Sweden than they are elsewhere. As noted by WHO "it is estimated that the rate of hospital use by older people is extremely high. Each inhabitant over the age of 65 spends an average of 16.5 days in the hospital each year. One might attribute this to insufficient resources for social housing such as old peoples' homes or retirement homes. This is not the case, for Sweden is especially well equipped from this point of view."

3. A Paradoxical Failure. A very active policy in favour of old people has been in place in Sweden. Development has occurred in both health and social spheres: numerous apartments and residences have been provided for the aged; programs of assistance and leisure activities have multiplied; a large number of long-stay hospitals have been constructed. But the special situation of the functionally limited aged has not been considered globally and has been rejected on the side of illness and the need for hospital care. Conceptions about aging and institutionalization factors had linked in a manner which had impeded coordination between the medical and social sectons. On the border of this situation however, there have already been numerous evidences of infiltration and some questioning is already occurring.

II. Toward an Improved Medico-Social Approach for Functionally Limited Older People

A. The New Orientation

Contrary to the situation in France one rarely finds the regulatory fever in Sweden which we display, nor is there the flood of circular letters that we unleash regularly on local authorities. Everything there is resolved at either the county or the communal level and there is scarcely any need for such machinery. But, as a result of this fact, developments undoubtedly proceed at a slower pace and in a more diversified way. Nevertheless the counties, which have regrouped as central associations, and the office of social development, have recently published several reports on the care of the aged which indicate new directions.

These reports confirm the fact that the system presents certain limitations. They are particularly critical about the lack of coordination between the communes and the counties and they indicate directions for the coming years:

1. Reinforcement of Primary Care. According to these reports the municipalities must have responsibility for organization of first line care: ambulatory care, home care, the day hospital, long-term care centers. These primary care centers must be organized around a perspective of people's mental, social and medical needs. The organization of care should be placed with a single administration and will bring into play physicians, nurses and physical therapists. Its development rests with health aides, construction of neighborhood care centers and medicalized local establishments.

2. *Emphasis on Maintenance in the Home.* One of the reports phrases this as follows: "to live in a familiar environment is more important than anything else for older people." This objective involves measures which require that every effort is taken to combat isolation and loneliness in older people. Neighborhood services must therefore be developed: Housing which is modern, available and adapted to need. If people are to remain at home the quality of the transportation system is considered especially important as is a good selection of shops. The reports add, however, that it is only if more personnel trained in health care services is employed in home care that sick and disabled people will be able to be cared for at home. The increase in the number of home care services must therefore go hand in hand with the services of home helps. Municipalities and counties must also cooperate more even if each continues to carry its own responsibilities.

The ideal model proposed is that of a committee for care planning which could divide the tasks and responsibilities between the communes, and teams of home care personnel, including home helps, nurses and health aides could ensure an ensemble of medical and social services in a geographic sector. This organization would be accompanied by systematic participation in funding between the municipalities and the counties.

If this problem were resolved it is probable that Sweden might rapidly and easily demonstrate its superiority to the French system: the status of physicians and nurses allows for coordinated organization since they are agents of the county whereas in France their private status frequently impedes the necessary cooperation. Additionally the reports emphasize the need to deliver the necessary services to the family: psychological support, provision for vacation respite care for the older family member, training in caretaking.

3. *Licensed Service Apartments.* In place of large boarding homes construction of small housing units and small service buildings integrated into neighborhoods is recommended. Alarm systems will be installed and day care centers will be

nearby. The usual size of apartments, two rooms, will be adapted to the needs of the functionally limited.

For some time to come, however, retirement homes will remain and will be occupied by very aged people. These will therefore be modernized and their method of operation must meet licensing with respect to social life and the autonomy of pensioners more closely.

4. Expansion and Transformation of Local Long-Stay Centers. According to plans established by the county, the number of long-stay beds must increase from 41,000 in 1977 to 55,000 in 1983—a growth of 33%. These establishments are reserved for people who have the most serious physical or mental problems but the duration of care in them is frequently very long. Therefore, long-term care centers should become living environments with improved provision for meeting medical need. Rehabilitation must therefore be developed in them in order that every possibility to increase autonomy is explored and every effort made to provide these long-stay services with the personal qualities of a home. The number of private rooms must be increased.

5. Care of the Senile. The development of senility may be prevented or delayed if efforts are made to avoid isolation and to encourage activities which have some meaning. For these people as well, the objective must be maintenance in their own homes for as long as possible. Day hospitals can be very useful in this effort.

When an institution becomes necessary it should be selected in a manner which avoids a later transfer; the majority can be served in long-stay facilities rather than in psychiatric hospitals.

Reports also stress the necessity for coordination of services and for intervention in all situations which must be oriented toward a systematic effort to transfer patients from institutions to ambulatory care. The discharge of patients from long-stay facilities will develop if rapid readmission in case of need can also be guaranteed.

Finally, the need for planning which will enhance coordination between municipalities and counties is re-emphasized.

Implementation of these objectives is based on the assumption that agreement between the municipalities and counties which is essential, will be established.

In contrast it should be stressed that, in France, the funding of such activities derives from medical insurance, and that its laws and regulations define the conditions of intervention: at the local level a prefectorial ordinance usually serves as the basis for expenditures from the fund. In Sweden there is no authority which can require expenditure of any kind from the localities; they are completely autonomous and politically responsible. One may therefore question the chances for success of these objectives: the maintenance of people at home, the increase of service flats, cannot avoid increased costs for the communes, and on the other hand they will reduce the costs to the counties since a certain number of hospital beds will no longer be utilized. The objective interests of the two partners are thus in opposition. And this, perhaps, is one of the explanations of the fact that the accent may be placed on medical establishments and not on the medicalization of social establishments. Perhaps the communes hope, as well, that health aides wil relieve the home helps of the responsibility for care of those who require the most attention.

These thoughts, however, neglect the fact that at least there does not appear to be the linkage of conflict and arbitration which characterize the functioning of our institutions in Sweden as there is in France. It is therefore probable that in the greater majority of cases the new directions which have been indicated will be followed because they are in the common interest.

Beyond the description of the general functioning of a system, this mission in Sweden allowed for a review of a number of practices which, while they may not be impressive in a large way, are nevertheless exemplary successes.

B. Some Additional Lessons

1. Some Technical Aids Which Support Autonomy. In addition to wheelchairs and other moving equipment, numerous small technical aids have been developed which support the autonomy of older people. The principle is generally a simple one since it is merely a matter of assistance with a function which is no longer possible because of physical limitations: A pincer on the end of a long rod so that objects can be retrieved without the necessity for stooping; forks and knives with special handles for rheumatic hands; special utensils for cosmetic care and for the kitchen. These technical aids are paid for by the county and are distributed without charge by the nurses in the sectors and by occupational therapists from long-stay hospitals. Studies which were made by the gerontological institute, however, indicated that in large part these aids are not used: because people are too ill; because they have not been taught to use them, or because they are too long or too short. The rehabilitation services are therefore teaching those people who are returning to their own homes to use this equipment in a training apartment in preparation for their return home.

2. Services Which Emphasize Readaptation. Two examples were particularly striking in the course of numerous visits:

The long-stay service at Kalmar (it is, in fact, intermediate stay) has its sole objective the discharge of the sick to their own homes: only 20% leave the service for a long-stay center. The others return home. This result is obtained thanks to the work of a team and the personality of a chief of service who considers that most older people are able to recover the autonomy necessary for discharge from the hospital, and to a system of home care developed by the hospital.

In a psychiatric service reserved for the aged the coordination of the work of the service team, in spite of the status of the people, emphasizes the will to restore the maximum autonomy. The symbol of this activitiy is depicted by a representation of a ladder of autonomy at the head of the bed where, each week, both accomplishments and regressions are recorded.

The service is divided into two sections in order to keep those who have retained some lucidity together. Evidence of the success of these activities was confirmed by the low turnover rate of staff caring for these people as opposed to experience in the majority of long-stay services.

3. Establishments Open to the Community. Whether they are residential institutions, hospitals, rehabilitation service, social or care activities, the programs are open to the population of the neighborhood or sector. In long-stay services a day hospital functions actively. Meeting rooms, shops for weaving or woodworking or gymnastics are open to older people in the community who often use them more than do the pensioners.

4. A very pragmatic research:

—The institute for Gerontology of Jonköping presents a special example in comparision with France, of work centered on polls and interviews with consumers.
—The National Institute for Research on Technical Material has launched studies of seven sections of the lives of handicapped people and of older people who are functionally limited: alarm systems, beds, chairs, nutrition. . . . It is a concern with research on the improvement of the details which make up daily life.
—This pragmatism in research on detailed adaptation is also found in the planning of buildings. The studies carried out by the service for planning and research of the counties (SPRI) indicates that the cost per bed in long-stay institutions remains stable as long as the number of beds exceeds 60. Competition has been undertaken for the building of a long-stay hospital. But, again differing from France it is their custom to allow newly constructed equipment to function for a while in order to analyze its faults so that errors will not be reproduced.

5. Organization of Active Groups of Retirees. Organizations of retirees do not limit themselves to the improvement of routines and the organization of public health services for their members. They also encourage participation in activities which provide retirement experiences which are really happy ones.

With respect to those questions which stimulated this mission, the present situation in Sweden was somewhat disappointing. If numerous and very interesting developments have been instituted with the initiative of the municipalities, in the area of the social services one must also conclude that the older person, just when he or she has need for care is rejected in specialized medical institutions whose medical administrators believe that in the majority of cases they will not be useful.

Nevertheless, and it is for this reason that we have emphasized them, the present arrangements have been analyzed and the new directions compared in their entirety with what is being tried in France. In this respect Sweden does not presently provide the example which it might have presented frequently in the past. It does, however, offer supplementary reference in a debate which is particularly difficult.

The fundamental lesson which is derived from this study is ultimately one which refers to institutions. The division of spheres of influence corollary to decentralization could, if they are not flexible at a given point, block all development. It is a question of clarifying the methods which impose coordination, or of clearing the way to unity of responsibility when several spheres of influence are concerned.

APPENDIX

SUMMARIES OF SEVERAL STUDIES UNDERTAKEN BY THE INSTITUTE OF GERONTOLOGY OF JONKÖPING

1. The Environment and the Functioning of Long-Stay Services (1978)

Results of a research study conducted by interview with sick pensioners in long-stay services; with those coming to the day hospital, and with personnel.

The study indicated:

—that pensioners consider it essential that long-stay services be close to their former housing
—that long-stay services should be constructed in older sections of the cities
—that the majority of patients are not opposed to large institutions
—that personnel consider the size of the service more important than the size of the institution
—that for the pensioners as well as for the personnel, the size of the room is more important than the size of the institution
—that people housed in the institution prefer to have meals served in their rooms, whereas those in the day hospital prefer a dining room
—that pensioners would like to have their rooms painted in attractive colors and would like to be able to bring their furniture and their souvenirs
—that they would like the doors of the rooms to have a window so that personnel could assure supervision

—that they would like an occupational activites room on each floor as well as one for the whole establishment

2. Future Long-Term Care in Sweden (1980)

The objective of the study produced by interview with pensioners in long-stay services and in retirement homes was to gather elements for the development of future long term services. The principal conclusions are the following:

—the majority of pensioners prefer to have long-stay facilities outside the city. However, the most dependent prefer to remain in the center of the city
—There was a general wish to have a park available and a preference for one-story buildings
—fewer than 10% of the pensioners would accept a four bed room and the majority want a private room
—personnel prefer that the services not exceed 20 beds
—People would like to bring their own furniture

Additionally a maquette was provided for their reactions: The "flexibility" which allowed, by a system of movable walls, the combining of two individual rooms, was considered excellent. The same was true of a grouping of rooms which permits personnel to work in teams. The absence of long corridors was also considered good.

The author concluded by wishing that similar inquiries might be repeated periodically with other people, particularly with families.

3. Organization of Care in a Long-Stay Psychiatric Service

The experiment consisted of using the same personnel for the same group of aged patients in order to reduce the number of people who provide information to the sick person. It was hoped that the mental confusion of these people would be reduced since they would have the opportunity of obtaining more precise information from personnel with whom they would feel secure and in whom they had confidence.

The "activation" of the sick rested primarily in the fact that they participated in routine tasks of the service: bed making, housekeeping, cooking and table setting. It was anticipated that increased attention would be paid to their own personal care: dressing and washing. . . .

On all counts the experiment appeared particularly convincing and this method of work has been recommended for all of Sweden.

Non-Institutional Long-Term Care in England, France and Sweden

Brahna Trager, ACSW, LCSW

Western European health care systems have not been considered seriously in the United States until relatively recently. The firm belief that the United States has the best health care in the world may have been partly responsible for this attitude, which has tended to discourage interest in either comparison or emulation. High technology, beautiful hospitals loaded with convenience and comfort for the consumer and with the latest and best equipment for the health practitioner support the image of a glossy, cure-oriented, successful industry. It would not appear that there is any need for curiosity or emulation except for certain emerging elements which have caused the image to darken. The best health care in the world does not appear to be producing the best results. Generally accepted indices compare the United States unfavorably with those of Western European countries. And for that relatively new section of the population—those in the older age ranges—there is a more marked impression that the quality of life, a rather vague but frequently stressed concept, is not as favorable for the older population of the United States as it is for the same population in Western Europe.

Brahna Trager is a health care consultant. She has prepared research studies in Home Care and Long Term Care and has participated in numerous projects related to non-institutional community care. She has administered medical care programs and home care programs. She is the author of three reports for the Special Committee on Aging of the United States Senate ("Home Health Services in the United States;" "Home Health Services—Current Status"; Adult Day Care and Related Facilities: A Working Paper"). She has also written texts for publication by the United States Department of Health, Education and Welfare ("Homemaker-Home Health Aid Services in the United States"; "Home Care in Chinatown—A Portrait in Health"). She is the author of "Home Health Care and National Policy," a special publication of Home Health Care Services Quarterly.

This article is based in part on a paper presented at the 110th Annual Meeting of the American Public Health Association, Montreal, Canada, November 14-18, 1982.

Unlike the United States all three of the countries, France, Great Britain and Sweden, which are the subject of this review, have had long standing, well developed, comprehensive social security systems. They differ in detail and in methods of administration; they are similar in the fact that, regardless of political parties in power, all three have established in their systems the assumption by government of responsibility for universal protection of the population from the major risks to economic security and health; the assurance of equality of access to such protection is a given.

Within the last three decades the need to plan effectively for a longer life span has stimulated a series of changes in their systems along with a great deal of forward planning for the population for which the life span has been extended.

All three countries have seen substantial increases in the proportion of older people in the populations, more marked in Europe than in the United States. The increase in Great Britain has been very sharp; in the ten year period between 1966 and 1976 there has been a 20% increase with most of the acceleration occurring in the older group (25.7% over the age of 75) so that the over 65 age group combining age 60 for women and 65 for men has reached 14%. Preliminary data for France in 1980 shows a similar level—almost 14% in the over 65 age range. For Sweden the increase is more marked. Sixteen percent of the population was over 65 in 1980 with more than 19% over the age of 80. These large increments in the extreme age ranges have important implications for planning.[1]

The principle of entitlement includes older people; age discrimination in services has stemmed less from moral judgements about personal responsibility than from misconceptions about the needs and expectations of older people. Experience and research together have changed previous assumptions about the kinds of environment older people prefer, about appropriate health care and about the process of aging itself. As these assumptions have begun to change, all three countries have been in the process of revising their systems of care for older people. The directions in which changes are being made differ from those in the United States since they start from an established base in which entitlement, service availability and access are key elements. Although these changes also differ in each of the three countries, depending upon the basic systems in which they have developed there is complete agreement in all three on one issue: this is expressed in the concept that care should be provided in the habitual environment, and if that is not possible, in a personalized environment which provides for maximum autonomy. The massive development of nursing homes for the elderly which has occurred in the United States has not occurred, nor is it being projected for the future in these countries, and the difference in the basic systems has not produced an industrialized approach in any of these countries.

Great Britain, as a first example, has had some form of social insurance since the beginning of the twentieth century. It was not until the introduction of the Beveridge Plan, characterized in the 1940's as "coverage from the womb to the tomb" that the National Health Service provided comprehensive care for the entire population. This comprehensive approach has provided access to the entire range of treatment and preventive services: community care provided by the family physician and primary care teams at the local level and hospital care provided in a system of different levels based on need and intensity. A chronic shortage of beds in acute care facilities both because of a lag in construction and increased use for longer periods by the chronically ill has resulted in a shortfall of beds estimated at 20%. The development of geriatric sections has only been a partial solution and there are differences of opinion about the quality of care in segregated facilities unless all of the diagnostic and treatment facilities are available.[2] The pressures have also made a necessity of the ideology that the home should be considered the optimum site of care wherever possible. It should be stressed, however, that the primary concern as it is expressed by English health professionals is not so much for costs as it is for improved care. The recognition that prolonged hospital stays, when they are not related to the need for treatment may have measurable negative results has stimulated a range of housing and community services which offer the prospect of reducing the pressure on institutions as well. It also reflects a growing concern for the quality of life for a population that does not in the main, resemble previous stereotypes about the aged. These developments had an initial advantage which is not present in the United States. It could be based on a community system of primary care in an organized pattern in which the family practitioner and the primary care teams composed of health visitors, visiting nurses, social workers, home helps (homemaker/home health aides) and related service staff could be made available on an as needed basis. Family physicians still make home calls. About 20% of all general practitioner consultations are for older people and two-thirds of these take place in the home when the patient is over 75 years of age. General practitioners receive weighted capitation fees for patients in the older age ranges (65 and 75). In 1975 over a million elderly people were treated by district nurses in their own homes or in general practitioner surgeries. They represented 42% of the total number of people served. About 15% of the cases visited by the health visitor are older people. The home help services which are considered "by common consent" one of the most valuable forms of practical support, provided about 90% of their service to older people in 1976; about half a million elderly people received the services.[3] Transitional treatment services have also been developed. These include geriatric day hospitals, usually attached to institutions; day care centers, which have received limited recognition and support in the United States have developed rapidly in England; more than 30,000 places were available in day care centers in 1976 and their numbers have been growing rapidly; this figure refers only to publicly funded facilities and does not include large numbers of places provided in the voluntary sector where it is estimated that upwards of a million people are cared for. The pattern in both the geriatric day hospital and the day care center is one which provides care during the day for an average of two days a week, although daily care may be provided. This care is supplemented in the home by the home help and meals service. Finally, a very wide variety of supplementary services is offered differing according to the need perceived by the local authorities and by local voluntary agencies. One report of a study of stroke patients identified approximately 180 different services, such as neighborhood warden systems, installed alarm systems, night sitter services, mobile laundry and bath services, equipment, chiropody, which is frequently offered as a basic service in the primary team as is special needs transportation. There is also a network of clubs for older people, many of them simple, but like the English pub they provide social contact and frequently function as the neighborhood information center.

The emphasis on domiciliary care has underlined the problems of housing for the older population. More than half of the housing occupied by people over the age of 60 was constructed prior to 1944, one-third before 1918. About 25% of the households headed by people over 65 lack at least one of the basic amenities (bath, hot water, inside toilets). The response to this need has been the construction of a variety of special housing facilities: Grouped housing with available central services, sheltered housing (with available warden services) and specially designed service flats. Public authorities have constructed about 190,000 units and 38,000 additional units have been provided through voluntary housing associations. Sophisticated call systems are being tried in lightly populated areas. In those units which are owner-occupied and old (about one-half of them pensioner occupied) insulation and remodeling are being provided along with increased heating allowances.

In spite of recent changes in Social Security which have improved the level of income for older people in England, income maintenance remains a real problem. Because of the complexity of some of the supplementary pension arrangements, it is estimated that about 50% of those who might be eligible have not applied, indicating a need for increased public information.[4]

A number of changes in the system of health and social services delivery occurred in 1974. Nevertheless the problems that remain are those related to the coordination of services. These originate in part because of the organization of the system with its different auspices and different levels of public and private responsibility. It is acknowedged that the need for home and community services is outstripping the supply; the need for additional acute care beds, may outweigh investment in the expansions of these services by government.[5] There is, however, a growing and vocal section of the voluntary community that will undoubtedly continue to press for the funding of community based care.

The French system of community service to its older population has developed somewhat more recently than the English system. In part this has been due to the strong family policy which has prevailed historically in France, and in part it is related to the complexity of the Social Security and Social Care systems which are based on benefits as a right but which tend to respond to need with categorical methods. Family policy has traditionally implied the family with children; the categorical approach usually means specific responses to specific needs as they arise, with the participation of the many mutual aid groups and associations in arriving at solutions, along with government.[6]

Planning and legislative action specific to the older population has accelerated in France since the 1960's although some action occurred as early as the late 1940's, particularly in housing. As in England and Sweden, concern has been related to the inappropriate use of hospitals by older people, particularly the very old. A more aggressive influence has also been felt in the pressures exerted by the mutual funds, the special associations and professional organizations which are so prominent in France. The terms "Solidarity, Social Justice and Equality" are more than rhetoric in France and these concepts have affected the approach to community care. The right of the individual to remain in his habitual residence, for example, was established by law in 1948. The older population has had access to medical care along with all other age groups, and older people have also participated in utilization of the extensive program of moderate rental housing which has been continuous until recently. Attention to the special needs of the older population, particularly those people who are economically and functionally limited, was made a "Priority Action" beginning approximately with the fourth five-year plan which was developed in the 1950's and thereafter this section relating to the elderly population appeared in successive plans. It is a more specific program, however, in the seventh plan[7] which was developed in 1977 and an even more active approach has been undertaken by the new government. The seventh plan projected increased income, a network of geographically accessible services intended to reach one-half of the approximately 270,000 older persons in need in order to avoid institutional placement and a program which would ensure that at least one million older persons would benefit from at least one of the group of projected community services. An increase in the pension base and a series of special supplements for such things as rent, assistance in moving, provision for reduced costs in restaurants and transportation was accompanied by certain mandated programs and several which could be selected optionally from a mandated group. The two basic services which were mandated were, first, a program of remodeling and adaptation of housing which had become dilapidated or which lacked the basic amenities. The second was the requirement that communities provide expanded leisure time and organized social activities, usually through the expansion of neighborhood clubs, for which provision had been made in previous plans. The plan also provided that older people might be removed for temporary periods from housing in severe climates or in isolated areas. The mandated services from which localities could elect to provide *at least one* service included the following:

> Preparation for retirement; expansion of the home help service (aides menageres); home care—the provision of medically prescribed home nursing linked with home help service; day care service on an experimental basis with care limited in eligibility and duration; a group of experimental services provided in centers, in clubs, in special group housing which would be more flexible than home nursing and less intensive and less costly than day care services. They would include such services as physical therapy, psychiatric care and general geriatric care. Special services such as a community telephone alert system, home delivered meals, congregate meals and exercise programs were also included as optional.

The mandated housing program projected the funding of about 20 housing units per year per sector with specific emphasis on the special needs of the elderly and the development of about 65 day care centers. The grouped services were projected for about 50 sectors. Certain of these services were already in place and funding was either supplemental or in the case of the newer programs, a form of "seed" money to assist local development. Implementation of this program was limited in funding and by the capacities of the local municipalities, although some elements of the program were implemented, primarily in urban areas.[8]

Concern for the elderly and the promise of action was a part of the election campaign of the Socialist Party and movement occurred almost immediately following the election. For the first time in French history there is a cabinet member for the aging in the Ministry of Solidarity. (The Ministry includes Social Security, Welfare, Immigration and Social Services.) The basic allotments of older people living on minimum incomes were increased in three stages over a two year period with increases amounting to about 42%. An active program is being undertaken with respect to establishments in which people are either being cared for or housed. It calls for the elimination of the oldest and poorest of the old people's homes, and for improvement of retirement homes which are inadequate; for "personalizing" long stay hospitals with the addition of social services and a more attractive physical environment, and, as a high priority effort, the provision of health services wherever older people are housed and are not receiving such care. The major thrust of the new program, however, will be the provision of additional services in the home. There have been about 150 home care programs in France providing services to about 3,000 older people. Funding will be increased so that this number can reach a first goal of 20,000 people in addition to the existing home help services provided mostly by mutual funds and voluntary groups which now care for about 350,000 elderly people. The salaries of home helps will be increased five-fold and training will be provided. The development and improvement of home care is also planned with the goal that the program will provide an average of 60 to 75 minutes of nursing care at home immediately following the prescription of a physician.

The stated theme of this effort has been the "socialization" of institutional care and the "medicalization" of home and community care. Housing policy, which has been continuous in France will be directed to grants for rehabilitation of older housing with the continued development of the very good specialized housing units (foyer-logements) which provide for grouped units in which people may live autonomously but which also provide excellent central services. Finally, because the entire program will involve decentralization 500 new field coordinators will be recruited and employed. Since the new administration can look forward to five more years in which to develop the program it will probably be implemented in phases with some dependence on the local communities which will now have considerable influence during the planning process.[9]

The relatively high level of services provided for the elderly in Sweden arises from basic, long established national policy concerning universal entitlement to what are considered the essential protections: income protection, access to health care, adequate housing, and supportive services necessary to an acceptable standard of living. Responsibility for these protections is assumed to belong to government and to extend to the entire population. The fact that the percentage of the Swedish population over the age of 65 in Sweden has increased from about 10% in 1950 to 16.4% in 1980 with further increases projected over the next 10 years[10] has accelerated the development of special programs for the aging population, among them adjustments in pensions and supplementary allowances, investment in a variety of innovative housing arrangements and changes in the traditional patterns of delivery of health and social care. With these there has been greater emphasis on avoidance of hospital care by increasing the availability of the community health-social support services.

Traditionally Swedish health care has been hospital oriented with a relatively high ratio of beds per population and a pattern of extended hospital stays. About 53% of physician visits take place in the hospital while about 30% are to the district physician within the primary care system.[11] These factors have stimulated the development in the 1960's and 70's of a variety of government provisions for home and community care: the issue of the quality of life also began to surface in the late 1950's with the development of a geriatric specialty in the health professions and the funding of specially adapted treatment facilities. In public statements there is now an emphasis on services to the aging which embody a set of principles in order to provide for "normalization" in life style and "to provide elderly people with a secure economic platform, good housing, an opportunity to obtain services and special care, and to maintain a sense of community with others in meaningful activities." This is a large view of government responsibility and while implementation has not been as global, there is no doubt that it is intended to be more than rhetoric. It is in the implementation of the first principle, that of "normalization" that the Swedish system has provided an innovative example of non-institutional care. The linkage which must exist between income maintenance, housing and health care is evident. Income maintenance for the elderly has been continuously upgraded since the late 1950's and changes in pensions for retired persons in 1979 have assured the possibility of almost a 50% increase over and above the basic pension plus additional allowances for housing, disability, for widowhood or earned income. The health and social care system provides additionally for services which maintain the elderly in the community.[12]

The services are very similar to those provided in England. Home care, which began to develop in Sweden in the late 1940's is provided by the municipality and includes physician care, nursing care, home help services, physical therapy, chiropody and aids and equipment. In 1980 about 41,000 older patients received home care services. Day hospital care, also similar to the English services, are usually attached to hospitals, clinics and local nursing homes. They are treatment oriented and are intended to offer services which may reduce hospitalization or to provide a post-hospital transition to the home. The pattern of care is also similar to the care in England; care for about two days a week combined with home help or home care. In 1980 there were about 4,000 places in day hospitals. There is, however, a projected increase to 52,000 over the next four years. In all of the community services there is consistent dependence on the home help services. Family members may be paid for this service but more than half of the care is provided by salaried staff, usually trained in approved programs. The home helps provide a total maintenance service; they may be assigned to nighttime care, or for 24 hour care. The municipality is responsible for the home help service and in 1980 almost 74,000 home helps provided service to 34,000 elderly people in addition to voluntary service. Supplementary services include mobile services such as meals, laundry, hairdressing and janitorial services as well as numerous locally developed services in the home.[13]

The housing programs in Sweden probably exceed in quality any system available to older people at the present time. The programs emphasize the importance of a comfortable living environment and housing standards are high. In addition to renovation of older housing there is a range of special housing arrangements: apartments for older people in ordinary buildings, small apartment groups with central facilities of which there were about 30,000 in 1980. The most interesting arrangement, however, is housing in multi-unit buildings which combine the features of an apartment, a hotel and a residential facility. They provide for complete autonomy along with full security and services as needed. They are usually located in urban areas. There were about 20,000 apartments in service buildings in 1980 and about one percent of people over 70 years of age live in them. An increasing number are being projected.[14]

The Swedish programs for the elderly are not without their problems. Aside from the difficulties of shifting from hospital-oriented care, there are recruitment problems because interest in geriatrics is limited among health professionals. The major problems, however, exist because of the different levels of responsibility for funding and service provision. The municipality must turn to the county for some services, the county to the region or the state. Easy service provision and coordination are not always possible.[15]

Nevertheless the movement is a forward movement and efforts to reorganize and integrate care are being made along with increased efforts to train professional personnel.

The conclusion that is inevitable when the service programs for the elderly in these three European countries are reviewed is that, while their programs may not immediately provide total solutions to the needs of their older populations, the direction which has been developed is based in the basic concepts of entitlement, equity and humanism. The older populations of these countries are not being expected to make do with rhetoric.

REFERENCES

1. Hobham, David. Great Britain. The Elderly all over the world. Monographs of the International Center of Social Gerontology, Paris, 1981; Old Age Care in Sweden. Fact Sheets on Sweden. The Swedish Institute, 1981; Annuaire des Statistiques Sanitaires et Sociales. 1981 (retrospectif 1970–1980) Ministère de la solidarité nationale. Ministère de la Santé. Paris, France.

2. Grimsley-Evans, J., Great Britain. In *Hospitalization of the Elderly. An International Perspective.* International Center of Social Gerontology. Paris, France, 1980.

3. Hobham, David. Op cit.

4. Ibid.

5. Grimsley-Evans. Op cit.

6. Schorr, Alvin. Social Security and Social Services in France. US Dept. of Health, Education and Welfare. Social Security Administration. Division of Research and Statistics. Research Report No. 7, US GPO Wash., 1965.

7. Programme d'action prioritaire pour favoriser le maintien à domicile des personnes agées ("PAP no 15"). Ministère de la Santé et de la Securité Sociale. Direction de l'Action Social. Paris, France (1976–1980).

8. Summary VII Plan–1976–1980. Ministries of Health and Social Action, January, 1977.

9. La circulaire "Franceschi" du 7 avril 1982 relative à la politique sociale et medico-sociale pour les retraités et les personnes agées. Ministère de la Solidarité Nationale. Secretariat d'état. Chargé des personnes agées.
Interview with M. Alain Gillette, Assistant Secretary to the Secretary for the Elderly, October 1981.
Aging in France: a new Policy. Information letter by the Secretary responsible for services to the aging, November 1981.

10. Just another age. A Swedish report to the World Assembly on Aging. 1982. The National Committee on Aging, 1982.

11. Old Age Care in Sweden. Fact Sheets on Sweden. The Swedish Institute, May 1981.

12. The Social Security System. The Swedish Budget 1982/1983. Summary prepared by the Ministry of Economic Affairs and the Ministry of the Budget, Stockholm, 1982.

13. Just Another Age. op cit.

14. Ibid.

15. Terroir, Patrick. Report of a Mission to review care provided to the aged in Sweden. *Home Health Care Services Quarterly,* Fall 1984/Winter 1984/85.

Economic Security and Old Age: French Perspectives

Alain Gillette

We are today facing a world in which the main concern in terms of social justice is not so much bringing to everyone a fair share in growth, but rather a fair distribution of cuts and setbacks.

To some degree, no region of the world, no kind of society, regardless of their diversity, has been spared. The fight against poverty, the fight for decent survival for all, well-being, self-respect is meeting head on with economic misman-agement and conflicting trends. So, as far as economic secu-rity for the elderly goes, the forecast for the immediate future is indeed not so bright.

This is what the United Nations report on the world social situation is telling us, while the U.N. General Assembly has endorsed the international Plan of Action adopted by 126 nations at the World Assembly on Aging in Vienna last Au-gust. The Plan of Action is the first comprehensive interna-tional document on the aging of individuals and societies, the first set of unanimously adopted recommendations on living and care standards for the aging. Here indeed is an ambiva-lent situation: a sharper knowledge of what policies on aging should be, but at a time of renewed economic and financial stress.

Two of the major recomendations of the International Plan of Action read as follows: Governments should "create or

Alain Gillette is a magistrate at the French "Cour des Comptes." Involved in gerontological field experiments and national planning for more than a decade, he was assistant-secretary to the Secretary for the Elderly in the French Cabinet from May 1981 to April 1983, and is now assistant-secretary to the Secretary for Family, Population and Migrants. 61-65 rue Dutot 75015, Paris, France.

This paper was presented at the Annual Congress of the American Public Health Association, Montreal, November 17, 1982.

develop social security schemes based on the principle of universal coverage for older people"; "Ensure that the minimum benefits will be enough to meet the essential needs of the elderly and guarantee their independence."

These fine principles are this morning's topics.

In such a field, oversimplification in so short a debate is inevitable. I shall not present technical answers, but rather raise some policy questions in, as I have been invited to do, a French and very personal perspective.

I shall first comment briefly on economic security itself, then refer to the international context, before discussing the major challenges that these first two points lead to, with respect to old age.

ECONOMIC SECURITY

What are we talking about? Economic security refers to a larger social security concept:

"Social Security" has a variety of meanings and scopes, involving social insurance, public assistance and publicly subsidized services. Overall, it involves a redistribution of resources, both among social groups and over the years, both for future use and current needs. Its goal is to safeguard individual economic security in the face of many personal changes and problems: health, maternity, invalidity, retirement. It is, today, an irreversible and major component of the social and economic systems in countries like France, where the labor market just would not work in the same way if it did not exist.

Let me make it clear that Social Security is not a luxury for the better years. It is an essential wheel of the French society and it could not back-track without a great deal of social and economic damage.

This does not mean that we should not endeavor to enforce cost-effectiveness and redeployment. In France, during the past 16 months we have spent more than three billion dollars on new improvements of old-age benefits. Some 2 million elderly of 61 years and older, one out of four, have seen their incomes, at the minimum guaranteed level, increased from 200 to 300 dollars a month, a 40% increase in real purchasing power. At the same time the purchasing power of some higher bracket citizens, earning 10 or more times that amount, will have eventually diminished by a few percent, because of payroll, income and capital tax increases.

This is what we mean by national solidarity, and within reasonable limits it proves to have a positive impact on the economy.

Some might say that the cost of the welfare state, whatever the degree of security it provides, has hindered economic progress. It is our conviction that it has worked the other way. Social Security, in every meaning, has been, in France, a major factor of growth. The quality of life it has enhanced also means a lot of industrial, housing and commercial expansion.

But, and this will be my second point, we are in the midst of an economic international crisis, where individual economic security is certainly at stake.

IN TIMES OF CRISIS

A little bit of history first: the modern industrial age, and here I quote the U.N. report, has "brought not only vastly increased wealth but also new forms of insecurity and misery to be mitigated, while some age-old problems affecting the welfare of individuals and social groups took on new dimensions."

Let us first have a look at the increased coverage.

Traditionally, work-injury coverage significantly came first; then sickness and maternity. And eventually old age, invalidity and death coverage. In 1950 only 54 countries had some old age, invalidity, death scheme. Today more than 124 do. At the same time schemes have widened their impact, and their cost has tremendously increased.

In 1960, Social Security was taking 9% of the gross domestic product of Western countries, and no figures were available for other parts of the world. In 1977, latest data available, the developed market countries have increased from nine to almost 17% their average gross national product share for Social Security. But on the other hand, since 1970 African countries have decreased from 2.8% down to 2.7%, Asian countries have increased from 3.5% to 4.5% and Latin America from 3.9% to 4.2%.

This means that while developed countries have almost doubled their effort, in a booming economy, developing countries can only afford one-fourth with slow expansion. Furthermore, while social insurance cash payments represent more than 60% of Social Security expenditures in developed countries, they represent less than 30% in developing countries, where in-kind services take the larger share. It is obvious that in those countries only a fraction of the population is covered by some social security scheme, in contrast with almost universal coverage in many developed countries. And while countries have in the past few years introduced or extended old-age coverage, these efforts have often been less than for unemployment.

The fact is that after two decades of almost full employment in developed market economies, unemployment has reached a level which has been so far considered unacceptable: more than 28 million people are unemployed out of a work-force of some 350 million. It is, of course, much worse in developing countries where, due to self-employment and family labor, statistics are not reliable; but low productivity, low, or no cash income, severe unemployment, are widespread.

This has several effects. One is that Social Security funding is deeply affected. Less employment, less national production and consumption, mean a lesser amount of receipts allocated to Social Security, whether through employer and employee contributions or special taxes and state participation. It also means higher cost for unemployment compensation. The result is a slowdown in Social Security extensions and increases.

This slowdown sometimes means a decrease in individual real income, in those countries where actual increase in purchasing power has recently come for most people not so much from wage raises, but through increased Social Security benefits, especially for the retired and the elderly.

And this occurs when, here again I quote the U.N. report on the world social situation, "1981 has marked the first year in a quarter of a century in which the *per capita supply* of goods and services failed to increase."

In many countries, the situation is therefore roughly that which *Time Magazine* pointed out in October 1982: "There is no secret about what must be done: either the payroll tax must be raised further, or some limit must be imposed on future (aging) benefit increases, or both."

The problem is that the economy cannot but suffer from either option, and that social justice is just as much at stake. It is important that we keep in mind both the situation of yesteryears, and that of other parts of the world: no economic security will be guaranteed in rich countries if the poorer countries keep getting poorer.

PERSPECTIVES

Let us envision some perspectives.

Retirement is obviously a major issue. There has been, for the past few years a significant lowering of the retirement age.

The world assembly on aging has insisted both on the right to work and the right to retire, noting that "age discimination is prevalent: many older workers are unable to remain in the labor force or to re-enter it because of age prejudice." It has recommended that "despite the significant unemployment problems facing many nations, in particular with regard to young people, the retirement age for employees should not be lowered except on a voluntary basis."

The problem is three-fold. On one hand, the right to re-tire early is a traditional demand from workers and trade-unions, and it is indeed a major social progress for those who have had unsatisfactory or tough working conditions and environment. On the other hand, the sometimes damaging consequences of being cut off from active society are well known. The cost of social or medical care due to loneliness and inactivity rather than age, should appear high if it were computed.

And finally, in the face of unemployment, there are strong pressures for earlier retirement in order to make room for the young unemployed.

There is no simple perspective to these questions: though it is obvious that one retiree is not necessarily replaced, unemployment is such that incentives toward earlier retirement are often politically welcome. Obsolescence of knowledge and skills is furthermore not always balanced by wisdom; let us face it. And in fact, many older workers have already chosen to retire several years before it is compulsory.

The answer should therefore be one of flexibility, opening options for everyone, and guaranteeing adequate benefits, even some financial neutrality in the choice. In France, costly guarantees have for some time been available, with an average of nearly 70% of the last activity income guaranteed for retirement.

Such a figure requires more than short-term financial balance. Structural questions are raised as well. The wisdom of having a large variety of retirement and superannuation plans is, for instance, questioned. This is a major factor in imbalance and inequity, although it has often been a good incentive.

One must bear in mind that economic security is not quite an insurance: in France one pays basically according to one's income and not in proportion to the risks covered, though most people have some kind of specific additional coverage. The basic guarantee, however, is against loss of income. This calls for a clarification of funding. In France, there is some talk about choosing between two clearer options:

—either a two or three stage system, with:
   1. a universal minimum guaranteed, with no welfare strings, or stigma, regardless of contributions,
   2. a second stage according to compulsory payroll contributions,
   3. a third optional, individually financed, stage.
—the other option would be a return to basic social security expectations,
   1. a universal and single contributive scheme,
   2. continuing the welfare non-contributive minimum benefits for all,
   3. and without specific advantages for superannuation plans which are today tax-free.

We are at present in an equivocal position and this is costly since some of the inequities must, in any case, be reduced through specific public funding.

No such effort can be undertaken, however, without a clear view of its effects on the economy, such as potential incentives or their absence, for manpower-intensive firms. The challenge is therefore not one of cutting down on expenditures, but rather of achieving a longer term balance, economically viable, socially equitable.

In these perspectives the question of what share of the national pie goes to economic security is a means, but not an end in itself. There is also the basic issue of demography, with the active/inactive population ratio. It is our view that demographic policy and long-term forecasts are a must if there is to be achievement, not only of economic expansion, but also of a better social balance and guarantee of the financial balance of the retirement funds.

This indeed requires a global analysis. The fact is that today longevity is more often achieved by the rich, culturally or financially, than by the poor. It reminds us that aging is a lifelong process, and that better economic security at old age may be an added injustice when security, either in health or labor, is not adequate at all ages. Risk factors with respect to the environment should, in this context be given emphasis and moderated accordingly.

With respect to health, let us again refer to the Vienna Plan of Action: "Existing social services and health-care systems for the aging are becoming increasingly expensive. Means of halting or reversing this trend and of developing social systems together with primary health care services need to be considered in the spirit of the declaration of Alma Ata."

The cost of health care has been increasing at a much faster rate than the economy, and there is growing concern that the possibility of checking this growth, at least without much damage, may be limited. Since the general trend has been that of a reduction of the share paid by the individual, the health care weight on social security and national budget is sometimes alarming. We should not, here again, forget that *per capita* health expenditures are 80 times less in the least developed countries than they are in the developed countries.

There is little doubt that comprehensive systems of compulsory health insurance are the only way to ensure some social equity in access to health care—the only way to guarantee that the elderly specifically, have a fair chance to receive adequate treatment without loss of dignity.

Very obviously, then, cost-effectiveness of the health delivery systems should be a major criterion in policy-making, assuming that the costs, and cost-effectiveness are really known. As the Vienna Plan of Action points out: "The trend towards increased costs of social services and health care systems should be offset through closer co-ordination between social welfare and health care services, both at the national and community levels. . . . all this must be done without detriment to the standard of medical and social care of the elderly." Home care and institutional care are "complementary to each other and should so link into the delivery system that older persons can receive the best care appropriate to their needs at least cost."

This is the policy we are financing in France now. Hospital costs are a good example. In France, as in the United States, they have recently increased two or three times faster than the general rate of inflation. Elderly patients account for up to half of the cost, while they represent only a tiny fraction of the aged population. Putting a lid on these costs is for developed countries an absolute necessity, though the numbers of beds and staff still vary widely.

France is approaching that problem through ending, in a year from now, a supposedly cost-based reimbursement system. An annual budgeting and programming system will instead lead to a sharper cost control, with responsibility in accounting.

Here again, we have proof that our debate on economic security requires far-reaching policies. Structurally, I would like to stress the impetus born in France from the creation of a cabinet position in 1981. The Department for the Elderly, with a secretary within the Ministry of Social Affairs and National Solidarity, has a significant impact on the development of a stronger and more coordinated policy on aging.

CONCLUSION

There are even wider choices to make. The well-being of the elderly, the health coverage, are of course only a part of today's way of life and way of death. The issues are also political and they call for political answers, both on a domestic and on an international level. It is up to each country to select and enforce its own options. But to some degree it is also the responsibility of the international community to reach agreements and commit itself to policies which would bring more security, economically and in other respects as well, to every human being. And this includes the International Division of Labor, trade agreements, and development policies for the third world.

Let me also state that world peace itself is both a stake and a means. For example, expenditures for military purposes have increased four-fold since World War II. They now reach more than 500 billion dollars a year, more than one hundred and ten dollars a year for every human being on earth, more than the annual incomes of hundreds of millions of them not to mention health and social coverage. And that provides one million times the Hiroshima bomb, among other armaments.

There is no simplistic answer to that challenge either, for the prevention of war is no easy task. But today's consumption, whether it is military or not, often competes with other priorities, and one cannot ignore the increasingly vehement reactions against what is termed an "armament culture." In that respect the future of social security is only one facet of a world in which national choices and international debates, or the lack of them, have widespread effects.

Thus, the economics of aging are basically a political issue, a global one, the outcome of which is not everywhere clear— and that is an understatement if one considers that while there were 200 million people aged sixty five and over in 1950, there will be six times that number forty years from now.

The countries gathered in the World Assembly on Aging did, quote: "Solemnly recognize," as a preamble, that "quality of life is no less important than longevity, and that the aging should therefore, as far as possible, be enabled to enjoy in their own families and communities a life of fulfillment, health, security and contentment, appreciated as an integral part of society."

We have many miles to go.

Report of the Expert Group Meeting on Long-Term Care of the Elderly and Disabled Organized by the International Social Security Association

Dorothy P. Rice

The charge to the participants at the Expert Group Meeting on "Long-term care of the Elderly and Disabled" made by Mr. Vladimir Rys, Secretary General of the International Social Security Association (ISSA) was to examine the role of social security in responding to the needs of beneficiaries for long-term care benefits and services, to look at the implications for the costs and financing of alternative social security schemes, to review the research on long-term care conducted by nations throughout the world, and to exchange information, knowledge, ideas and experiences in this area. The group considered 11 reports and after 2-1/2 days of open discussion of the excellent papers prepared for the meeting, the participants had fulfilled the charge very well. Facts were presented, issues were raised, questioned, and discussed. Ideas were challenged; consensus was reached on some issues while agreement on others was not reached.

The ISSA Secretariat divided the theme into three main topics which will be followed in this summary report:

Dorothy P. Rice is Professor, Aging Health Policy Center, University of California, San Francisco.

This paper is adapted from the concluding remarks made by the author, who served as general reporter for the meeting held on June 20–22, 1983 in Oslo, Norway.

1. Identification of long-term care needs;
2. The role of social security in meeting long-term care needs; and
3. Research on long-term care.

IDENTIFICATION OF LONG-TERM CARE NEEDS

All of the papers highlighted the changing demographics and their impact on long-term care needs in which the aging of the population throughout the world will result in a rapid rise in the near future in the number and proportion of the population that will be elderly. Every nation, be it industrialized or less-developed, recognizes that as more people live longer, chronic illnesses causing limited or total disability and functional dependency, will create burdens and multiple needs for the individual, family, and society. These needs transcend social security and encompass many sectors of economy, including income security, medical care, housing, social services, transportation, education, and recreation.

Both the public and private sectors are deeply involved: Social Security cash allowances, welfare, and private pensions given to the entitled recipients provide income support to maintain a degree of independence and choice of services for individuals who require limited long-term care services. Medical, social, housing, and transportation services for these individuals may be supported and provided by private insurance and/or government programs. All levels of government are often involved: federal, regional, state, and local community resources.

The general parameters of the population at risk for long-term care were presented in terms of population projections by the United Nations and by individual nations by age and sex based on assumptions of continued decline in death rates, control of formerly fatal infectious diseases, continued advancements in medical technologies and therapies, and improvements in life styles. According to United Nations data on projected population growth, people aged 60 and over will be the fastest growing population group in the world and will number over 1.1 billion by the year 2025, representing more than a 5-fold increase in the 75 year period between 1950 and 2025. During this same period, the world's total population will increase only 3-¼ times from 2.5 to about 8.2 billion persons.

As a result of current high fertility and low mortality rates among the younger ages in developing nations, their age structure will significantly change. By the year 2000, 61 percent of the 590 million elderly in the world will be in developing regions; this proportion will increase to 72 percent by 2025. In terms of actual numbers, there will be more than 2-½ times as many aged in the less developed regions than in the more developed ones. The implications of these statistics are sobering in view of the relative lack of services, facilities, and skilled health personnel to care for these people who are at risk for long-term care in these regions (Rice). By taking advantage of the innovations in the industrialized world, such as vaccines, antibiotics, and microbiologic techniques, developing countries have achieved much faster rates of improvement in health status than those achieved in Europe and the United States over a longer period.

There was general consensus that to plan social insurance and other programs to meet the long-term care needs of the aged and disabled, precise methods and detailed data are needed. To estimate the long-term care population in policy relevant terms requires that the the total population at risk be disaggregated according to the probable use of alternative modes of long-term care services as a function of personal and long-term care system characteristics. Moreover, for purposes of projecting long-term care needs and use, it is necessary to understand the transitions in the use of various modes of care as a function of changes in the population and the system.

Model building, incorporating dynamic macro- and micro-level perspectives, and utilizing a cohort approach, was suggested as a strategy for developing a fuller understanding of long-term care needs. This is a complex task requiring a multiplicity of data collection and analytic strategies. Perhaps the most complex task, however, is to bring the diverse sources and types of information together to estimate behavioral relationships among the various components, such as health status, marital status, financial resources, social networks and supports, housing and living arrangements, geographic distribution, public policy, and technological innovations (Luce, Liu and Manton). Societal implications of long-term care are sufficient to justify long-range investment in data collection and analysis. Adequate differentiation also must be made in identifying the special and differing needs of the two separate population groups—the disabled and elderly populations.

Various definitions of long-term services were developed by the participants. There appeared to be general agreement that to address the multiple and varied types of needs of the long-term care individual, services must cross the boundaries between income maintenance, health, social, personal and domestic care, and housing and transportation services.

Although there is no consensus in the literature regarding the proportion of aged who are likely to be in need of long-term care services, it is estimated that approximately 10 to 20 percent of the aged population are in need of some form of care at home, in the community, or in institutions (Morginstin and Shamai). This estimate refers to an entire range of supportive services such as short-term health care, residential homes, sheltered housing, rehabilitation and other social services, but does not include care provided informally by the family. Furthermore, this estimate is based on the actual use of services and therefore is not a reliable indicator of absolute need, nor of the level of need for services. Both of these factors must be taken into account in planning and estimating long-term care needs and the cost of a long-term care program.

It was recognized that needs create programs that in turn create new demands that impact on projections. Supply and demand for social services and benefits are determined by factors and developments which often have nothing to do with the schemes themselves. The overriding goal of long-term care expressed by all was maximum possible functional independence to assist the disabled and aged individuals to continue living in the community, provide services which meet their needs, and provide a continuum of care as their level of independence changes.

THE ROLE OF SOCIAL SECURITY IN MEETING LONG-TERM CARE NEEDS

The main charge to the participants was to examine the role of social insurance in meeting the long-term care needs of the elderly and disabled. There was healthy discussion relating to this broad subject area. Basic questions were raised:

1. Can social insurance programs meet the long-term care needs of the aged and disabled?
2. Can a social insurance program be designed to encompass the needs for income support as well as for services in kind?
3. Are there trade-offs between traditional social security cash benefits and new service benefits?
4. Are social security pensions a right not to be tampered with, reduced or changed?
5. Should social security pensions be reduced when individuals are institutionalized and their daily shelter, food and maintenance, needs are being taken care of?
6. Should savings be taken into consideration in payments of benefits?
7. Will cash allowances or service benefits reduce voluntarism, the role of the family, and social networks and links in meeting the long-term care needs of the elderly and disabled?
8. Can incentives be designed to encourage the appropriate use of long-term care benefits without creating an increase in demand for services?
9. Can a social insurance program be designed to develop protection not only when an individual is institutionalized, but when he or she lives in the community?
10. What are the criteria for prioritizing the needs and benefits for long-term care?
11. Are the long-term care needs of disabled workers different than those of the elderly?
12. Do the high rates of unemployment conceal the needs of disabled workers wherein marginal workers with some disability become totally disabled because jobs are not available during a recession?
13. Is the division of authority between health, social services, and social insurance agencies a barrier to accomplishing the goal of providing services to meet the diverse long-term care needs of the elderly and disabled?
14. How can the individual or the family requiring assistance be helped in the face of a confusing array of agencies and professional personnel each with its own organizational structure and professional ideology?
15. How can political considerations of resource con-

straints be balanced against the real long-term care needs of the elderly and disabled?

16. Has sufficient emphasis been placed on prevention to reduce future long-term care needs?

17. What are the appropriate roles of federal, regional and local community organizations or authorities in the provision of long-term care benefits?

The range of questions outlined above may leave the impression that no answers, solutions, or alternatives were presented and discussed at the meeting. On the contrary, the wide and differing experiences of countries represented at the meeting were most illuminating. Following are illustrative examples and are not meant to be all inclusive.

Canada (Charron)

Several relatively recent developments have occurred with respect to health care for Canadian seniors that assist in meeting many of the long-term care needs of the elderly: (1) the development and implementation of a universal, first-dollar health insurance system; (2) an emphasis on preventive health to avoid the occurrence or to minimize the extent of functional dependency among the elderly; and (3) the implementation of alternatives to institutional care, including an array of home-based services and programs that promote a sense of self-esteem and dignity and provide mental stimulation. Such programs include crisis centers for the depressed, lifestyle enrichment programs, safety hazard identification, monitoring and visiting services, day care, meals-on-wheels, homemaker and educational services.

Suitable housing that provides privacy, is close to neighborhood amenities, and has facilities for socialization, is crucial to the physical and well-being of the elderly. Also needed are low rental units, home maintenance programs, as well as a variety of financial incentives for the elderly to remain in the general community including reverse mortgages, reduction or elimination of property taxes, reduction of fuel and utility costs, home adaptation and repair grants, and interest free loans for home renovations.

Increased income security, accessibility to medical services and low-cost rental housing have permitted the Canadian elderly to stay in their own homes longer than they otherwise would. The primary goal is to help the elderly continue living in the community, provide services which meet their needs and provide a continuum of care as their level of independence changes.

Israel (Morginstin and Shamai)

Legislation enacted in 1980 created a long-term care insurance branch under National Insurance to formulate guidelines concerning the goals, scope and contents of long-term care insurance. The intent of the law is not to substitute for, or finance, existing formal services, but to complement the existing system of service provision by making available additional resources to the disabled aged individual and his family as well as for service development.

A considerable amount of data on the demographic characteristics of the aged in Israel has been compiled and analyzed. Research has been undertaken on home and community services. Findings show that most aged persons in need of assistance in personal care and household maintenance receive such services from the family, while only a small proportion receives help from organized formal services in the community. The implication is that a gap exists between absolute needs and coverage by formal service agencies, and that the principal service provider is the family. In terms of long-term care insurance, it may be expected that a good proportion of aged who will be eligible for benefits on the basis of functional disability will have access to families who can provide care either directly, or will be able to obtain the necessary services in the community. The conclusion is that cash benefits will be an effective instrument in assisting the eligible disabled aged individual and his or her family by covering part of the costs incurred in providing or obtaining services. For those who have no family, who receive insufficient services from family, or who are unable to obtain services independently, it will be important to directly provide services in kind via Long-term Care Insurance.

Scandinavian Countries (Walmann)

Old age pensioners' right to retain income during stays in Scandinavian health institutions is the subject of this paper. Denmark, Norway, and Sweden have varying provisions for retaining income and property during stays in hospitals and long-term health care institutions. In all the Scandinavian countries, stays in public hospitals are free of charge for pensioners for an initial period. In this "free period" the pension is paid at the same rate as if the person were not in an institution; the length of the "free period" varies from country to country.

After the expiration of the "free period," a stay in a health institution has financial consequences for pensioners who must pay for the stay or accept full or partial stoppage of their pension. In Sweden the pension is the same whether the pensioner is in a health institution or not, and consequently the pension can be used in the same way as any other income to pay for his or her stay in an institution. However, in Denmark and Norway a stay in an institution affects the actual pension right or the size of the pension paid by National Insurance. Whether actual pension rights should be reduced (as in Norway and Denmark) or whether pensions should be unaffected by a stay in an institution (as in Sweden) is a debatable question. Further, in Denmark and Sweden, the pensioner's property is not taken into account in stipulating the level of payment during institutionalization; in Norway, property is not exempt. The latter approach may lead to problems when the pensioner assigns the property to others.

Federal Republic of Germany (Oldiges)

In the Federal Republic of Germany, the elderly age 60 years and over comprised 19.4 percent of the total population in 1980 and an additional 9 percent were disabled. A great variety of protection and assistance provisions are available to the elderly and disabled. Included are the sickness, accident, and old-age insurance, self-help from relatives and neighbors, self-help groups and charitable organizations, and assistance from public authorities and social insurance organizations. Occupational and medical rehabilitation, including emphasis on guaranteed employment and vocational training, have become important elements of care for the disabled.

It is estimated that 50 to 80 percent of long term care is currently met through social assistance. Based on an analysis of needs, many different activities are necessary in order to maintain treatment and care and especially the social integration of the elderly and the disabled. On humanitarian grounds alone, community care services must take priority over institutional care so that the further development of social service centers is of special importance in the Federal Republic of Germany. Possible solutions under consideration to the problem of the creation and financing of community and institutional care include changes in old-age and sickness insurance, as well as the introduction of special insurance to cover long-term care based on the principle of solidarity. There is agreement on that such a system should cover both institutional and community care.

Poland (Radzimowski)

The projected changes in the nation's demographic structure and the erosion of the caring role played by the family present increasingly serious social policy problems in providing appropriate living conditions and in organizing life for the growing number of people over retirement age. Taking into account the variety of needs, social welfare organizations provide four basic types of assistance: cash benefits, benefits in kind, social services, and assistance from the former workplace.

On January 1, 1983 a general reform of the old-age, invalidity and survivors' pensions came into force. All types of pensions are covered by the reform, including those for workers, for independent farmers, for war disabled and survivors, and for minors. As a result of the reform, the system of old-age, invalidity and survivors' pensions became universal and were also synchronized with earnings. This is a very important feature of the reform because it enables the retired and the disabled to share in the rising national income on the same basis as the economically active population. Cash allowances also are provided to all those aged 75 years and over to cover some of the costs of long-term care.

France (Coudreau)

In 1980, 14 percent of the population were aged 65 and over; projections indicate this proportion will increase significantly in the future, affecting the level of sickness insurance expenditures. Although care in a medico-social or health establishment is indispensable as the aging process advances, most elderly persons are in sufficiently good health to want to remain in their own homes. To obtain this objective, a network of home-help and domiciliary care services, particularly social services, has been created.

Domiciliary care services were covered by sickness insurance beginning in 1978, and amended in May 1981. Payments were made directly by the funds in the form of fixed daily rates to cover the cost of nursing care, nursing auxiliaries, massage, physiotherapy, and pedicures. Under the 1981 decree, the only costs covered are those for nursing care, or nursing auxiliaries; all other services are excluded. Such services may be provided to anyone over 60 years of age without prior approval; they may also be provided to people under age 60 but, except in cases of emergency, prior approval is required from the fund's medical adviser.

The development and financing of domiciliary care under sickness insurance will make it possible to avoid the transfer of the elderly to long-term care establishments and to avoid unjustified hospitalization. Although it is recognized that the program has improved the health care of the elderly who prefer to stay at home, there are difficulties in controlling costs of the program within budgetary limits.

Netherlands (DeGier)

Under guiding principles of distributive justice, a wide range of social welfare provisions in addition to social security benefits have been created to meet the needs of the elderly, sick, disabled and the handicapped. Both the supply and the demand for social services and benefits are determined to a large extent by factors and developments that have nothing to do with the schemes themselves, such as demographic, economic, medico-technological and social-cultural factors.

In addition to pensions, provisions have been made for

accommodations for the elderly (adapted dwellings, rent re-
bates, old people's homes, etc.), provisions for family care,
residential and non-residential health care (hospitals, nursing
homes, physiotherapy, district nursing, etc.), and provisions
in the socio-cultural, recreational and community fields (old
people's passes, credit cards for public transportation, etc.).

Provisions for long-term care for the disabled, handicapped, and long-term unemployed in the Netherlands also
have been developed. The increasing numbers of persons receiving benefits will continue to place financial strains on the
social security system. New policies to deal with these problems demand that the trade-off between social security and
economic efficiency has to be reviewed and scrutinized.

United Kingdom (Winterton)

The Government's current policies and administrative arrangements for meeting the needs of the elderly and disabled
people are aimed at enabling them to lead full and independent lives in the community, preferably in their own homes.
In order to achieve this goal, both health and social services
authorities are looking at ways of increasing community-based
support. The hospital services are concentrating increasingly
on the assessment of patients' needs, the treatment of acute
and chronic conditions and the provision of rehabilitation to
enable the majority of people to return to their homes as
quickly as possible. Where disability, frailty or social circumstances preclude remaining in or returning to the community,
care is provided in a residential or nursing home or long-stay
hospital. Efforts are being made to create a more domestic
atmosphere in these institutions and to give residents more
control over their own lives.

Research on long-term care is funded from a number of
sources: the central government, in particular the Department
of Health and Social Security and the Department of Environment, the Medical Research Council, the Social Science
Research Council, universities, local health authorities, and
several larger charities. Research has focused on studies of
residential care, including a survey of 400 homes to provide
information on residents, staff, and the homes; a survey of
local residents to identify potential volunteers and their ac-

ceptance by the staff; and a survey of local authority homes to assess the reactions of elderly residents and staff to their physical surroundings.

Research on community-based long-term care included a survey of supporters of confused elderly people in the community and the establishment of experimental schemes to support elderly people in their own homes by bringing together packages of care suited to their needs. It is essential to relate research findings from a wide range of sources in such a way that they can be used in policy development and to disseminate them widely.

United States (Rice)

Long-term care services for the aged and disabled in the United States encompass a wide variety of programs, institutions, organizations, and personnel supported and financed through government and private funds. Medicare, Medicaid, Social Services, and the Older Americans Act all provide services for the aged and disabled, but they differ in benefits, eligibility, financing, and administration:

1. Medicare, Title XVIII of the Social Security Act, enacted in 1965 and amended in 1972, provides health insurance coverage for the elderly and disabled. The Medicare program is federally administered and financed from Social Security employer and employee payroll taxes, general revenues, premium payments, deductibles and copayments. It covers hospital care, physicians' services, limited nursing home care and home health services.

2. Medicaid, Title XIX of the Social Security Act, enacted as a companion to Medicare in 1965, provides matching funds to states to finance medical care for low income persons who are in families with dependent children or who are aged, blind or disabled. Under federal guidelines, the states have the discretion to develop eligibility standards, benefit coverage, provides qualifications, payment schedules, and administrative structure. About two-thirds of Medicaid spending are in behalf of the aged and the disabled.

3. Social Services, Title XX of the Social Security Act, established in 1974, authorized payments to states for a wide range of community social services for individuals and families. The program is directed in part to particularly vulnerable populations such as the aged and disabled young persons. The program goals call for the maintenance of economic self-support and self-sufficiency and preventing or reducing inappropriate institutional care by providing community-based care, home-based care, or other forms of less intensive care. Types of services covered under this programs include homemaker services, preparation and delivery of meals, transportation, counseling, adult day care, and supportive health services.

4. The Older Americans Act of 1965, reauthorized in 1978, funds an array of services for persons age 60 and over. The Act established a network of state and area agencies on aging to plan for a comprehensive and coordinated delivery system for social services for the aged, such as information, referral, homemaker services, transportation, nutrition education, counseling, research and demonstration projects, and training.

Despite the availability of a vast array of health and social services, families and friends still provide the bulk of long-term care services to the aged and disabled in the United States. A major issue in the delivery of long-term care services is the design of the Medicare and Medicaid programs which reimburse for the most costly institutionalized care. In response to the rising concern over the cost, appropriateness, and the quality of care provided in institutional settings, the Federal government is encouraging the development of alternative community-based services and evaluating methods to reform and integrate long-term care health and social services.

RESEARCH ON LONG-TERM CARE

A variety of research activities and findings were presented at this Conference; research proposals that emerged are summarized below:

1. Identification of Long-Term Care Needs

Research is needed in defining the population at risk for long-term care, differentiating between the younger disabled persons and the elderly. Isolating the determinants of long-term care and model building, incorporating data from multiple sources as well as longitudinal data, are essential components.

2. Assessment Technology

Procedures and instruments for systematic evaluation of elderly and disabled persons are needed to provide a basis for identifying treatable conditions and for recommending interventions and sources that are rational, beneficial, humane, and cost-effective. These assessment technologies are also essential for planning, administration, and financing of such services.

3. Evaluation Research

Various demonstration projects in long-term care are undertaken, especially experimentation with alternatives to institutionalization. Evaluations of these programs should be carefully designed utilizing control groups, if possible, and taking into account all costs while maintaining the quality of care provided.

4. Research on Outcomes of Care

Research on the efficacy of clinical and social therapies is necessary to enable rational choice between alternative approaches. Such research must carefully consider specific subgroups at risk. Research is needed in the following areas:

a. Ways that assessment protocols can assist in clinical management decisions in long-term care screening, diagnosis, monitoring, and prognosis. Are different types of assessment protocols needed for different roles?
b. Tests of reliabilty, validity, and usefulness of these assessment instruments must be undertaken. How can these instruments identify and assess the needs for long-

term care in terms of chronic medical treatment, physical and mental functioning, social supports, and environmental characteristics?

c. Use of standardized assessment for aggregated data in management and planning decisions about long-term care. Can these tools be used instead of or as a supplement to clinical judgement?

5. Costs of Long-Term Care Services

The rising cost of institutional care has resulted in several studies of the costs and cost-effectiveness of care delivered in alternative settings. Some studies indicate that alternatives tend to become additions to existing services and the additional costs tend to outweigh savings from reduced institutionalization. This experience is apparently replicated in Europe, where ready availability of home based services may not reduce institutionalization. Additional research is needed to determine the extent to which the availability of formal support services retards institutionalization without destroying the informal support network and its willingness to provide care.

6. Prevention and Health Promotion

To avoid the occurrence or to minimize the extent of functional dependency among the elderly and disabled, research is needed on the effectiveness of specific preventive services and programs for the elderly, such as screening for chronic disease, pre-retirement counseling and nutrition education. The possibility of preventing the onset of illness rather than treating diseases may reduce future long-term care costs while improving the quality of life.

7. Manpower Training

Training of appropriate manpower for the care of the elderly and disabled is an operational as well as research issue. The deficiencies in services of the wide range of health personnel involved in long-term care are well known, although not emphasized in the Conference. At all stages of the long-term care process, involvement is needed of physicians, trained nurses and nurse's aides, medical specialists, therapists, dentists, nutritionists, social workers, recreation workers, and others. Basic to improvement in the education of health and social service workers and the staffing of all types of long-term care services are: (a) the development and regular recording of information on the needs of chronically ill, disabled, and aged patients, emphasizing functional status and the nature of disabilities requiring assistance; (b) comprehensive medical-nursing-social evaluation of patients to determine appropriate placement and treatment; and (c) methods of classifying patient data to establish staffing requirements and patient needs.

8. Building Long-Term Care Components into the Social Security System

Research and demonstrations are needed to examine trade-offs between Social Security cash and service benefits to meet the long-term care needs of the elderly and disabled while controlling the long-range costs of social security programs.

CONCLUSION

The issues and potential solutions to the problems of long-term care for the elderly and disabled were presented and discussed during the course of this Conference. Perhaps more questions were raised than answers provided. Policy analysts throughout the world recently have focused attention and concern on the needs of the aged and disabled populations. There is a need for more research into various aspects of the long-term care process, the organization, delivery, costs and financing, and the evaluation of national policies adopted to meet these needs. In this research Conference, we learned from our respective national experiences and hopefully moved forward toward meeting the long-term care needs of the elderly and disabled and improving the effectiveness of the services provided.

REFERENCES*

Charron, M. "The Impact of Demographic and Social Trends on Long-Term Care Needs of Canada's Elderly."

Coudreau, D. "The French System of Domiciliary Care for the Elderly."

DeGier, H. C. "An Overview of the Dutch System of Long-Term Care of the Elderly and the Disabled."

Gilliand, P. "Domiciliary Care: A Partial Alternative to Institutionalisation."

Luce, B., K. Liu, and K. Manton. "Estimating the Long-Term Care Population and Its Use of Services."

Morginstin, B. and N. Shamai. "Planning Long-Term Care Insurance in Israel."

Oldiges, F. J. "Long-Term Care of the Elderly and Disabled in the Federal Republic of Germany."

Radzimowski, Z. "Methods of Alleviating the Effects of the Economic Crisis on Pensions for the Elderly and the Disabled in Poland."

Rice, D. P. "Long-Term Care of the Elderly and Disabled: Introductory Report."**

Walmann, B. "Old Age Pensioners' Right to Retain Income During Stays in Scandinavian Health Institutions."

Winterton, P. "Research into the Long-Term Care of Elderly People in the United Kingdom."

*Papers presented at the International Social Security Association Expert Group Meeting on "Long-Term Care of the Elderly and Disabled," June 20–22, 1983, Oslo, Norway, and published in *Long Term Care and Social Security*, International Social Security Association, Studies and Research No. 21, ISBN 92-843-1018-0, Switzerland 1984.

**Published in the *International Social Security Review*, Number 3, 1983, pp. 299–326.

Toward a Social Policy on Caring for the Aged in Israel

Miriam J. Hirschfeld, RN, DNSc

INTRODUCTION

There is an ancient and time honored Jewish tradition of caring and mutual responsibility—caring and responsibility of the individual for the group and the group for the individual. Beliefs, ideologies and responsibilities are remembered, but how can they be translated into social policy, a social policy of caring which must be at the heart of planning dependency care? How can the responsibility of care for the dependent elderly in the home be divided between the individual caregiver, the family and the State and who shoulders which part of the actual caregiving burden?

Israel is a modern state with a rapidly growing population of dependent old people and very limited resources. In this article, I shall first describe some factual information necessary to grasp our context of dependency care and then some of our trials and errors in developing a system of long term care. Finally, I shall quote some ideas on caring and tending, which we hope one day shall reflect a social policy of true mutual caring between the individual and the group, the person in need and the State.

HISTORICAL AND DEMOGRAPHIC TRENDS

The population of Israel comprises indigenous Jewish and Arab populations, augmented by Jewish mass immigration from 104 countries following the creation of the State in 1948. The age, sex and ethnic structure has thus undergone considerable change over the past 35 years. The total population in

Miriam J. Hirschfeld is Lecturer in the Department of Nursing, Tel-Aviv University and National Coordinator for care of the aged and chronically ill, Kupat Holim, Sick Fund of the General Federation of Labour in Israel.

1981 was 3.9 million made up of 3.3 million Jews and 640,000 Arabs (Moslems, Christians and Druze). Within the Jewish population, the proportion of elderly was 3.7% in 1950, rose to 9.7% in 1980 and is expected to reach 10% by 1990. The proportion of elderly within the non-Jewish community has decreased as a result of the high Arab birth-rate and a significant decrease in child mortality from 5.4% in 1950 to 3.1% in 1980, to a projected 2.8% in 1990. The absolute numbers rose from 9,000 in 1950 to 20,300 in 1980.

Of the 338,000 Jewish elderly only 4% were born in Israel; 70% immigrated from Europe and America, and the remaining 26% came from countries of North Africa and Asia. The elderly population is itself aging. The old-old represented 28.6% of the aged in 1950 and 31.1% in 1980. They are expected to comprise 40.1% of the elderly by 1990. The overwhelming majority of the aged (95.6%) live in the community in private households and 92% live in urban areas.

Over 80% of the elderly live in family situations, 43.8% are elderly couples and 37.8% live with other family members. This percentage is falling gradually. About a fifth, mostly women, live alone (Chartbook on aging in Israel, 1982; Israel National Report to the U.N. World Assembly on Aging, 1982).

In the last decade service provision has undergone a profound change. The early years of the State demanded immediate solutions on a mass basis. This did not allow the time or resources for a range of solutions or a special service system. The major responsibility for the aged was shifted to absorption authorities and to Malben, a voluntary organization, which mainly developed institutional settings. As the influx of immigrants decreased, the emergency passed and with the introduction of National Insurance payments to the elderly in 1957, there began a gradual quest for the development of a range of long-term care services for all population groups (Bergmann, Habib, & Tomer, 1980).

OLD PEOPLE IN ISRAEL—WHO ARE THEY?

Three major groups constitute Israel's aging Jewish population: (1) the veterans, (2) those elderly who arrived after 1948 from the Islamic countries and (3) those who arrived after 1948 from Europe (Hirschfeld, 1982).

The Veterans

The veterans are a generation of pioneers. Their ideas, beliefs and hard labor laid the foundation of today's Israel. They are the people who dried the swamps, who built the roads, who worked in the desert and who built cities from the sand. Many of them contracted the infectious diseases endemic to the Middle East. They believed in hard physical labor and in the rebirth of an old nation. And they idealized youth—old age was not part of their mental imagery. They foresaw many complex needs of a growing and changing society, but most of them did not foresee that aging would be a factor to be dealt with—neither on a personal, nor on a societal level.

The Elderly from the Islamic Countries (Oriental Jews)

There is a small, but highly cultured and well established veteran population of Oriental aged from families living in Israel (Palestine) for many generations. But the majority of Oriental elderly immigrated from Asia and Africa in the years following Israel's Declaration of Independence (1948).

With large variations within this Oriental group, there are nevertheless common features as compared to the European group. The leadership and government was patriarchal and religious, daily life was dominated by religious practice and law. There were large extended families. The level of education was usually low (most of the women and about one third of the men were illiterate) and since Jews were not allowed to own land in Arab countries, there were no farmers. Most of these immigrants were artisans or petty traders and very few were professionals.

It was difficult for the older men to become integrated into the Israeli labor market. Migration led to changes in their social status, which were often reflected in status change within the family. While the deep cultural and religious ties helped many to adapt, despite great adversities, others found refuge in the dependent role of chronic illness (Miller, 1965; Weihl, 1972; Shuval, 1963, 1970).

The Elderly from Post War Europe

Four hundred thousand to 500,000 survivors of direct and prolonged Nazi persecution have come to Israel after WW II. These numbers include those who spent the war years in flight or captivity, hiding in forests or under false identity, enslaved in labor gangs, starving in Ghettoes, or condemned to death in concentration camps equipped with gas chambers, where only one out of 600 survived. The literature (Lederer, 1965) describes survivors as suffering from the "persecution syndrome": anxiety, chronic depression, insomnia and nightmares, voluntary social isolation, inability to forget, haunting guilt feelings and a wide array of physical after-effects: headaches, dizziness, peptic and duodenal ulcers, hyperthyroidism, vascular diseases, cancer and organic brain damage.

One of the characteristics of these after-effects is that they do not diminish over time; aging exacerbates the symptoms. Many of these survivors face their old age with severely limited physical and psychological resources.

In summary, while an unprecedented amount of cumulative stress characterizes many of Israel's old people, the hope of a new beginning and the shared faith that "we must find a way," lends an involved urgency to our caring trials and errors.

THE ISRAELI HEALTH CARE SYSTEM

Ninety-six percent of Israel's population are insured in one of four sick funds, with Kupat Holim of the General Federation of Labor as the major fund, covering 83% of the insured, including 95% of the Jewish and 71% of the Arab elderly. Kupat Holim was founded long before the State and developed a strong primary care base with 1250 neighborhood clinics in every single urban area or agricultural settlement. Preventive and curative care is the major responsibility of the salaried nurses and physicians, but in recent years these community clinics have developed home care. During the course of a year about 19,000 patients (most of them elderly) receive home visits. Nurses perform 65,000 such visits per month. While Kupat Holim either provides or completely covers ambulatory care and acute hospitalization, the needs for homecare are far from adequately met. The aging of the population has been paralleled by the tendency of young families to move to the suburbs, so that today in the inner city clinics, up to 45% of the members are aged 65 and over, while the newer suburban clinics have even less than 5% in that age group.

The elderly account for 50% of all clinic visits and for 30% of all bed-days in acute hospitals; their hospital admission rate (per thousand) is more than double as that for non-elderly. The average duration of hospital stay for the aged is twice as high than for younger people; 40%–60% of most hospital departments are occupied by those 65 and over.

The above hospitalization statistics encourage the notion of "bed-blocking" or unnecessary stay of elderly in general hospitals (Bendel, 1983). Ageism often precludes a critical evaluation of the potential for recovery of old people, which exists despite the intensity and complexity of health conditions, given high quality and adequate duration of treatment and care. The bed-blocking argument tends to discredit the need for both hospital care, as well as intensive home care services and leans toward demanding more beds in cheaper long-term care institutions.

The Ministry of Health is the other major health care provider with responsibility for preventive community care, acute and long-term hospitalization.

LONG-TERM CARE

As most Western countries, Israel is dissatisfied with her long-term care system. There are several major issues which must be addressed: (a) insufficient home care and community services; (b) high use of institutional services; (c) low quality of much of institutional care; (d) insufficient psycho-geriatric services; (e) insufficient family counseling and relief services; (f) unequal geographic distribution of services; (g) a rapid rise in total long-term care expenditures, borne primarily by government revenues; and (h) limited availability of funding, due to budgetary constraints.

In August 1980 the Israeli Knesset passed the Nursing Care Insurance Law, which promises the coverage of long-term care needs to every citizen. The Minister of Labor and

Social Affairs appointed a public commission to formulate the principles (i.e., kind and range of services covered, eligibility criteria and organization of services) of this law. The commission was comprised of 22 members appointed either to represent a body or organization with impact upon services to the aged and chronically ill (e.g., the Ministries of Health, Labor and Social Affairs, and Finance; the trade unions (Histaadrut); Industrialist Organization; Kupat Holim), or appointed for their professional expertise (nurses, social workers and physicians).

The plenary commission subdivided the task finding into four subcommittees: (1) services desired, (2) existing services, (3) rights and eligibility criteria, and (4) organization. Each of the subcommittees submitted their reports in writing to the plenary sessions of the public commission where details were discussed in an effort to reach unanimous recommendations.

The staff of the National Insurance Institute and of the Brookdale Institute of Gerontology and Adult Human Development in Israel performed the research necessary to provide the sub-committees and the commission as a whole with the necessary data. The Law will not and cannot replace the current system of long-term care services, but it is hoped to strengthen them by guidelines for service development, as well as by providing sources of financing.

In the summer of 1981 a survey was conducted to describe and analyze the existing long-term care services (Factor, Guttman & Shmueli, 1982) as one of the major research efforts toward the implementation of the new Law. The study covered two major types of services: (a) institutional services: homes for the aged, hospitals for the chronically ill, acute and rehabilitation geriatric wards and (b) community services: services delivered at the elderly's home (nursing care, personal care, etc.); day care services delivered in central community facilities; housing services; and cash benefits for purchase of home appliances, mechanical aids and other special needs.

The final recommendations of the commission were split (Nursing Care Law Report, 1983). The majority report recommended the provision of long-term care services as a national insurance scheme (need, but not means tested), while a minority report asked for the funds to be channeled to the budget of the major service providers, who would then be responsible for developing and providing services, without having the funds linked to an individual insurance scheme.

The question of allocating funds to the development of institutional versus home and community services was heatedly debated. The final resolution calls for a fifty-fifty division of development funds, where home care services have priority in the "community care bracket" and improving the quality of nursing care beds has priority in the "institutional care bracket."

Nearly a year has passed since the commission submitted its recommendations, but neither payments to individuals, nor provision of services have begun yet. There is mounting social and political pressure to begin the distribution of the badly needed accumulating funds.

HOME CARE AND OTHER COMMUNITY SERVICES

For each shekel (Israeli currency) spent on formal community care, the long-term care system spends more than five shekels on institutional care. Division of responsibility between the health and welfare sub-systems (Welfare Regulations No. 4.3, 1973) is the defining characteristic of the home care and community service system. The health sub-system has responsibility for those aged who are "nursing" patients. The criterion seems to be confinement either to bed or the house. For the "nursing" aged the health sub-system has responsibility for medical, nursing and personal care, while domestic care, nutrition and transportation remain the responsibility of the Ministry of Welfare. The Ministry also has full responsibility for those elderly who are not home-bound.

Responsibility in the health sub-system is divided between Kupat Holim and the Ministry of Health on the basis of a well-defined agreement (Kupat Holim Circular No. 3/80). Kupat Holim is the agent responsible for providing care.

At the time of the Yom Kippur War (1973) Kupat Holim suddenly realized how ill-prepared the primary health care clinics were to care for all the bed and home-bound patients who were discharged from the hospitals in order to make beds available if needed for the wounded. In each health area a health care team was established consisting of a physician, nurse, social worker, physiotherapist, occupational therapist and secretary. The team provides only direct services to the patient whenever the primary health care team is unable to do so. The responsibility of direct care remains in the hands of the family physician and nurse. The role of the team is:

1. To evaluate the needs of the patient and family to-gether with the primary care team;
2. When necessary, to instruct and give consultation to the primary care team in the care to be delivered;
3. Arrange for the solution of social problems;
4. Provide physiotherapy;
5. Arrange for occupational or speech therapy;
6. Arrange for home maker and personal care services;
7. Deal with other agencies such as the Ministry of Health, Ministry of Welfare for coordination of fund-ing for patient care;
8. Arrange for institutionalization should this become necessary;
9. Arrange for day hospitalization (which is still a scarce commodity);
10. Obtain equipment for the patient such as wheel chairs, walkers, and special beds.

During the course of a year the home care teams serve 5,000 to 6,000 patients and there are always about 3,500 on the active lists. There are about 12,000 to 13,000 additional patients receiving home care by the primary clinic team (Zackler, Shavit, & Boroshak, 1979/80; Kupat Holim Circular No. 105, 1983).

Also within the government health services there has been a growing involvement in services to the elderly. The estab-lishment of a Division of Chronic Illness and the Aged in the Ministry of Health is but one expression of this trend. More recently the reorientation of Maternal and Child Health Clin-ics to Family Health Clinics with a built-in preventive care element for the aged (including home visits) gives evidence to the expansion in nursing services to the aged.

The welfare sub-system organized casework in the majority of local welfare offices along an integrated case load model, i.e., the aged constituted a part of the worker's load of families and his/her care. Another model gradually emerged. Special case loads of elderly were dealt with by special workers. This "categorical" approach became the officially preferred model. This development was paralleled at the national level by formalization of the "Service to the Aged" desk/division at the Ministry of Welfare. In 1978 this ministry merged with the Ministry of Labor to become the Ministry of Labor and Social Affairs (Bergmann, Habib, & Tomer, 1980).

Eshel, an inter-agency organization for the development of services to the aged, bridges the health and welfare subsystems. Eshel develops services where national government, Kupat Holim and other sick funds, municipal authorities, and local voluntary organizations cooperate on providing comprehensive service at the neighborhood level. Eshel is also active in developing manpower and financing demonstration projects. One example is the "categorical" approach of nurses stationed in either the Kupat Holim or governmental Family Clinic and being responsible for providing home-care in a given neighborhood. It is too early to judge this model's effectiveness.

Habib (1980) raises specific questions regarding the adequacy of present home-care arrangements.

1. Problems arise from the division of responsibility and the need of the aged and their families to approach several addresses. The basis for assigning persons to the various categories is vague and leaves room for needy persons to be denied eligibility by both subsystems.

2. The responsibility of the Health and Welfare Ministries does not extend to fully *guarantee the supply* of home care services, but rather focuses on financial support in their purchase. While the health care network takes major responsibility for the supply of the medical and nursing components (most clearly for those insured in Kupat Holim), the supply of personal assistance is left either to the voluntary Matav organization or to unorganized agents within the community. These are valid sources, but they are not necessarily available in all areas or for all the elderly in need. Nursing home-care is also in very limited supply, since it is not part of the Kupat Holim insurance scheme. It is a benefit developed through force of circumstances, rather than covered by policy commitment. While Kupat Holim realizes the overwhelming need for

providing intensive home-care, financial restraints keep her hesitant in extending this service according to the needs.

Thus, despite the provision of financial support for nursing, personal and home-maker services, supply limitations limit actual access to these services. In addition, the financial support becomes insufficient at our present rate of skyrocketing inflation (approximately 200%/year).

3. A third defining characteristic of the home care system is that the responsibilities of both the Ministries of Health and Welfare are limited by the *available budget.* In the Ministry of Welfare this is a function of each local agency's budgetary situation. This seems different from the situation with respect to institutions, where there is budgetary responsibility to provide a place for all those deemed in need, or at least a spot on the waiting list.

The welfare sub-system has strictly defined the maximum amount of support and the requirements for participation by the aged person in meeting the costs (Welfare Regulation No. 4.8, 1979). Criteria have been defined in the health sub-system for the extent of personal aid and those who should receive it. Conditions for financial participation have not been defined, since Kupat Holim is hesitant to apply means-tested users charges. The basic principle guiding the development of Kupat Holim since 1911 was that each member pays according to his ability and receives services according to his need.

In summary, the rising need for home care is faced with three major constraints: the organization of a universally integrated service, the guarantee of high quality supply and the financing of home care services. Great hopes are set on the Nursing Care Law (discussed above) which will have to address these questions and find badly needed solutions.

THE FAMILY AND OTHER "INFORMAL AGENTS"

High costs, budget constraints, and perhaps also the difficulty of providing home care services responsive to such a wide variety of needs have led policy makers to seek reliance on "informal agents" for support of the elderly. While there is a genuine and justified concern in maintaining elderly persons in their natural community environment for as long as possible, there is an urgent need to critically assess the capacity and willingness of informal support networks to be *the* viable support to the very impaired.

In Israel, as in other countries, the family is the major source of services to dependent members. But despite extensive helping patterns, a demographic dilemma (Treas, 1977; Brody, 1981) does confront kin networks: (a) increased life expectancy, especially for women, which is often accompanied by prolonged dependency; (b) increased life expectancy for the very disabled due to effective treatment of intercurrent conditions and the development of medical technology; (c) declining fertility rates–fewer younger family members are available to share the responsibility of support; (d) increased geographic mobility; and (e) economic developments. A growing number of young and middle-aged women must choose between nursing frail parents, or working to support their families. This demographic dilemma is of particular significance in Israel, where (a) because of historical circumstances and immigration patterns approximately 12% of the Jewish elderly have no living children and another 9% have no children living in Israel (the figures are based on a one percent representative sample of Jewish urban non-institutionalized persons aged 65+) (Weihl, Nathan, Avner, 1970; Weihl, 1983); (b) there is a steep increase in the old-old, which means that the elderly community is itself growing older; (c) acute care and medical technology have developed way and beyond long term care services, and (d) yearly inflation has risen to over 200% which increases the need for women to be gainfully employed.

In a recent study of 181 families caring for severely impaired aged and 92 families caring for severely impaired children in Central Israel (Hirschfeld & Krulik, 1984) the tremendous resilience of these families was documented, but also the severe burden they were shouldering. But while we know that many families in fact do nurse their frail relatives at great physical and psychological cost, we also know that other families are unable or unwilling to do so. In addition we do not know what can be expected of families and other social networks, who have not yet been faced with the necessity and choice of caring for a dependent old person.

Shuval, Fleishman, and Schmueli (1982) have shed some

light on this issue in a recent study of the informal social support of 652 elderly in Baka, a Jerusalem neighborhood. One of their questions was network resiliency, which they defined as the ability to continue providing support for the elderly person in the future when greater needs are likely to occur. The findings showed that elderly persons tended to be more pessimistic than their primary helpers about the likelihood of support in the future. However, both the elderly person and their helper agreed that sharing a home and giving financial assistance were the most difficult and showed the least resiliency, while short-term personal care and listening to problems are the easiest. Resiliency decreases with increasing demands (time, effort and money) put upon the network's resources. Networks which have developed habits of support are likely to continue this pattern when increased needs arise. However, those which have not been active supporters in the present or recent past are unlikely to become active in the case of increased need. The affective quality of relations is a significant predictor of resiliency.

The results also indicate that there is a "hard core" (60%) not prepared to live with the elderly person under any circumstances. However, the remaining 40% would likely show increased readiness in response to assistance for building an extra room and personal care assistance for the elderly person. Cash payment was perceived as the least effective encouragement.

In light of the above facts informal agents do not seem to be the panacea for the problems arising from the increased needs for dependency care. No doubt that families and even friends and neighbors will continue to play an important role in the care of the dependent elderly, but their efforts must be met by those of the health and social care systems.

CONCLUSION

In his lecture on *The State of Care,* Roy A. Parker (1980) distinguished two usages of the term "care": The first, the idea of caring about, of concern and moral involvement and the second, the direct work which is performed in looking after those who cannot do so for themselves. This second active and personalized manifestation of care in feeding, washing, lifting, protecting, representing and comforting, he called *tending.*

To translate a moral heritage of mutual caring and responsibility between the individual, the group, and the State into a modern reality, I do believe we must accept the challenge Parker so clearly defined: "to design and implement social policies for tending which do four things:

1. Reflect and incorporate a general social concern for the dependent—'caring about.'
2. Reduce the inequalities between those who tend and those who do not.
3. Secure high standards.
4. Respect the sensitivities of the dependent and not consign them to the role of burdensome fellow human beings." p. 31

For years the notion of "ein breira"—the Hebrew words for "no other choice"—was used to explain Israel's tenacity in face of great adversities. It seems to me that the challenge of answering to growing numbers of dependent human beings has become another "ein breira" if we want to preserve a vital aspect of Jewish pride and moral heritage.

REFERENCES

Bendel, J.P. *Bed blocking in general hospitals by elderly patients waiting for post-discharge arrangements.* Jerusalem: Joint (JDC) Israel Brookdale Institute of Gerontology and Adult Development in Israel, 1983, D-95-83.

Bergman, S., Habib, J., & Tomer, A. *Manpower in services for the aged in Israel.* Jerusalem: Joint (JDC) Brookdale Institute of Gerontology and Adult Development in Israel, 1980, D-45-80.

Brody, E.M. The dependent elderly and women's changing roles. *Mount Sinai Journal of Medicine,* 1981, 48(6), 511–519.

Chartbook on aging in Israel. Brookdale Institute of Gerontology and Adult Development in Israel, Jerusalem, 1982.

Factor, H., Guttmann, M., & Shmueli, A. *Mapping of the long-term care system for the aged in Israel.* Joint (JDC) Brookdale Institute of Gerontology and Adult Human Development, 1982, S-15-82.

Habib, J. *Toward the next decade of long-term care services for the aged in Israel.* Joint (JDC) Brookdale Institute of Gerontology and Adult Human Development, 1980, S-4-80, Jerusalem.

Hirschfeld, M. *Primary health care and the elderly in Israel.* Paper prepared for the INI Conference on Innovative International Nursing approaches in primary health care of the elderly. Project Hope, Millwood, Va., June 7–10, 1982.

Hirschfeld, M. & Krulik, T. *Family caregiving over the life cycle.* Tel-Aviv University, 1984, Unpublished Research.

Israel National Report to the U.N. World Assembly on Aging (Vienna, 1982). *Aging in Israel,* Jerusalem, 1982.

Kupat Holim Circular No. 3/80, Agreement of Kupat Holim and the Ministry of Health on the participation of Kupat Holim in payments for home care. (Hebrew).

Kupat Holim. *Demographic-diagnostic characteristics of patients under care of the Kupat Holim regional home care teams on 31. 12. 1981,* No. 105, February 1983, (Hebrew).

Lederer, M. Persecution and compensation. *Archives of General Psychiatry,* 1965, 12(5), 464–474.

Miller, L. *Social change and mental health in Israel.* Paper presented at the Samuel Rubin International Series Lecture of the Postgraduate Center for Mental Health, New York, January, 1965.

Nursing Care Law Report. *The commission for suggestions of guiding principles toward the nursing care law.* Presented to the Minister of Labor and Social Affairs, Jerusalem, May 1983 (Hebrew).

Parker, R.A. *The State of Care.* The Richard M. Titmuss Memorial Lecture 1979–80, Joint (JDC) Brookdale Institute of Gerontology and Adult Human Development, S-3-80, Jerusalem, 1980.

Shuval, J.T. *Immigrants on the threshold.* New York: Atherton Press, 1963.

Shuval, J.T. *Social functions of medical practice.* San Francisco: Jossey-Bass, 1970.

Shuval, J.T., Fleishman, R., & Shmueli, A. *Informal support for the elderly: Social networks in a Jerusalem neighborhood.* Joint Israel. Brookdale Institute of Gerontology and Adult Human Development, Jerusalem, November 1982.

Treas, J. Family support systems for the aged: Some social and demographic considerations. *Gerontologist,* 1977, *17*(6), 486–491.

Weihl, H. Selected aspects of aging in Israel: 1969. In D.O. Cowgill, & L. Holmes (Eds.), *Aging and modernization.* New York: Appleton-Century-Crofts, 1972.

Weihl, H. *Changes in family structure of the aged and their inter-generational relations over a period of twelve years.* Final Unpublished Report, Brookdale Institute of Gerontology and Adult Human Development in Israel, Jerusalem, 1983.

Weihl, H., Nathan, T., Avner, U., Finkelstein, N. & Getter, N. *Investigation of the family life, living conditions and needs of the non-institutionalized urban Jewish aged 65+ in Israel.* Ministry of Social Welfare, Jerusalem, 1970.

Welfare Regulations No.4.3. *Distribution of roles among the Ministry of Health and Ministry of Welfare, Ministry of Labor and Social Affairs,* Jerusalem, April 1973 (Hebrew).

Welfare Regulations No.4.8. *Ministry of Labor and Social Affairs,* Jerusalem, October 1979 (Hebrew).

Zackler, J., Shavit, N., & Boroshak, Z. Care of the home bound patients. *Kupat Holim Yearbook,* 1979/80, *6,* 49–58.

The Continuation of Home Care to Severely Impaired Children and Aged in Israel: Family Attitudes

Tamar Krulik, RN, DNSc
Miriam J. Hirschfeld, RN, DNSc

ABSTRACT. There are a growing number of children and aged with severe chronic health problems in the community. Mothers become the prime caregivers to these children and aging spouses or middle-aged offspring the caregivers to these aged. The services offered to these families are determined by economic and social conditions, as well as changing fashions, rather than knowledge of the patients' and caregivers' needs. The purpose of this study was to assess the impact of homecare upon families caring for children versus those caring for aged and these families' attitudes toward continuation of home care versus institutionalization. The families included in the study were drawn randomly from the case load of community nurses in central Israel.

In-depth interviews were conducted with 92 families of severely impaired children and 181 families of severely impaired adults and aged in their homes. While the majority of both populations carry a heavy burden of caregiving over years, they also receive gratification from their ability to care for their patient at home. There is little difference between those caring for children and those caring for adults in their attitudes toward continuation of home care.

Mental rather than physical impairment, a deteriorating illness trajectory; depression, aggression and tension of the care-

---

Tamar Krulik is Lecturer, Department of Nursing, Tel Aviv University, and Pediatric Clinical Specialist, Sheba Medical Center, Israel. Miriam J. Hirschfeld is Senior Lecturer, Department of Nursing, Tel Aviv University, and National Coordinator, Care of the Aged and Chronically Ill, Kupat Holim, Sick Fund of the General Federation of Labour in Israel.

This paper is based on research project, "Family Care Giving to Severe Chronically Ill Children and Aged." This research was partially supported by the Schreiber Fund, Sackler Medical School, Tel Aviv University.

283

giver, the absence of sufficient social support and home care services correspond with negative feelings toward continued home care.

The perceived impact of caregiving responsibilities upon the caregivers' lives, the ability to tolerate and manage symptoms and above all the quality of the patient-caregiver relationship influenced the caregivers' attitudes toward institutionalization in both populations. Family attitude toward continued home-care and institutionalization of children and adults are compared and the needs for services discussed.

INTRODUCTION

In Israel, as in other developed countries, we are witnessing a profound socio-biological change which creates a new reality described by Isaacs et al. (1972) as the "*Survival of the Unfittest.*" Large numbers of human-beings (children and aged) survive for many years in a state of complete dependency. Increased longevity and the sophistication of medical and nursing interventions have led to a situation where many very impaired old people survive for many years. Some are cared for in institutions, but the majority are cared for by their families—usually middle-aged and old women. A similar process has taken place in regard to children. Large numbers of multi-handicapped and severely impaired children live to adulthood. Most of them are cared for by their parents, mainly their mothers in the home.

The services offered to these families are determined by economic and social conditions, as well as changing fashions. While "the only right way" used to be institutionalization of a very dependent person, this has changed to home care as "the only right way." These fashions are of course largely dependent upon the above mentioned economic and social considerations. A major objective of our study (Krulik & Hirschfeld, 1984) was to provide at least some basic information on the impact and meaning of home care for children versus home care for aged. In this article we shall focus upon the variables influencing families' attitudes toward institutionalization versus continued home care. We hope that this knowledge will add some "objective" substance to our health-care services fashions.

STUDY METHOD

Data were gathered from the main caregiver in home interviews, using a structured questionnaire which covered different aspects of home care, along with demographic, disease variables and availability of professional and social resources. Indexes for cost burden, symptom/behavior tolerance and management ability, and social support were constructed. These indexes were based on previous research (Krulik, 1978; Hirschfeld, 1978) and indicated adequate reliability (Alpha Cronbach).

STUDY SAMPLE

The study sample consists of 181 families caring for adult and elderly and 92 families caring for children, all Jewish. The criterion for inclusion in the study for both populations was that the impaired person had a disease or disability for which institutional care was an option.

One hundred and eighty-one principal caregivers to chronically ill or severely impaired adults were interviewed in their homes. The families were chosen randomly from lists of homebound patients cared for in primary health care clinics of Kupat Holim (Sick Fund of the General Federation of Labor) in central Israel. Approximately 95% of the population in this age group is insured through Kupat Holim in Israel. One hundred sixty caregivers were interviewed by nurses and the rest by social workers. All families approached agreed to take part in the study. The interviewers were trained. Data were collected in 1981–82.

Ninety mothers and two sisters who were the principal caregivers to chronically ill and severely impaired children were also interviewed in their homes. The families were chosen randomly from lists of chronically ill and severely impaired children identified by public health nurses in government family health clinics also in central Israel. Approximately 80% of the children in Israel receive preventive and follow-up health care in these clinics. The 92 caregivers were interviewed by nurses who were trained for this assignment. All families but one which were approached agreed to take part in the study. Data were collected in 1981–82.

DEMOGRAPHIC VARIABLES OF PATIENTS
AND FAMILY CAREGIVERS

Impaired Adults

Of the aging population, 97 were male and 84 female; their ages ranged from 36 to 98 with a mean age of 70.5 and a mode of 72. They came to Israel from 22 countries of origin with the bulk from Eastern Europe, about 17% from Asia and Africa, and only 4% born in Israel. Most of the sample came from urban areas and only approximately 4% from rural settlements. These demographic variables are similar to the trends of the aging Israeli population at large. Socio-economic status was defined according to the patient's occupation most of his/her life; 3.3% were defined as low-low, 21% as medium-low, 58.6% as middle, and 17% as high-middle. National statistics suggest that 25–30% of Israel's elderly are in an economically comfortable position, and that economic stress is significantly correlated to requests for institutional placement (Israel U.N. Report, 1982). This study sample might be slightly better-off economically than the national average.

Impaired Children

Of the sample of children, 54 were male and 38 female. Their ages ranged from one year to twenty years; 50% were 6 years and older. Sixty-three percent received their education in institutes for special education. All children and adolescents were born in Israel. All subjects came from intact families.

Caregivers for Impaired Adults

In the sample of those families caring for adults 125 caregivers were female and 56 male (84 wives, 48 husbands, 33 daughters, 4 sons, 2 daughters-in-law and 10 others). Their ages ranged from 24 to 89, with a mean of 65 and a mode of 82. The caregivers' countries of origin were similar to those of the patients' except with a greater proportion (12%) born in Israel. More than a third of the caregivers had only one child or no children at all; about half had two or three children; and 13%

had four children or more. Four percent were illiterate; 35% had only elementary school education; 45% had been in secondary school, and 15.5% to a university. About one-fifth of the caregivers were gainfully employed, and 30 caregivers reported that they did not work because of their caregiving responsibilities. The socio-economic status of the caregivers is similar to that of the patients. 39% defined their families as non-religious, 43% as traditional, and 18% as religious.

Caregivers for Impaired Children

All 92 principal caregivers for children were female (90 mothers and two sisters). Their ages ranged from 22 to 50 years. Thirty-five percent of the mothers were born in Israel (primarily to European parents); 45% came from Asia and Africa, and 20% came from Anglo-Saxon countries. Forty-two percent of the mothers finished only elementary school; 27% finished high school, and only 2% took some studies at the university. Their professions were mainly within the lower status groups, e.g., secretaries and skilled workers. The majority of the mothers (75%) were not gainfully employed; many reported that they had to give up work or plans for work because of the child's condition. The socio-economic status of these families was within the middle to low groups. These mothers were all caring for other young children besides the sick child (15% had four or more other young children). Twenty-eight percent defined their families as not religious, 48% as traditional, and 24% as religious. All but one family resided in a metropolitan area.

DISEASE-RELATED VARIABLES

Impaired Adults

In the population of impaired adults, each subject had up to five diagnoses (in order of declining frequency): heart disease 38.9%, cerebrovascular disease 35%, hypertension 29.4%, orthopedic and rheumatoid disease 29.4%, diabetes mellitus 28.9%, organic brain syndrome 25.6%, chronic lung disease 13.4%, partial blindness 12.8%, cancer 12.2%, depression 11.1%, and Parkinson's disease 10.6%.

Impaired Children

The children in this study had multiple handicaps, mainly related to the central nervous system. (This is not surprising since only these diseases are socially accepted as a reason for institutionalization of the child—see criteria for inclusion in the sample). In the sample there were, in declining frequency, 52.2% children with severe motor and mobility problems, 47.8% with severe retardation, 28.3% with cerebral palsy, 19.5% with minimal brain damage, and 10.8% with severe convulsive disorders.

Physical and Mental Impairment in Total Samples

Since both groups (adults and children) represented many different diseases, for comparison purposes they were divided into three main categories of impairments:

1. Patients with physical impairments which included 61.8% of the elderly and 30.4% of the children.
2. Patients with mental or emotional impairments which included 7.3% of the elderly and 27.3% of the children.
3. Patients with both physical and mental impairments which included 30.7% of the elderly and 41.3% of the children.

ACTIVITIES OF DAILY LIVING
IN IMPAIRED ADULTS AND CHILDREN

The degree of help needed (independent, partial help sometimes, partial help always, complete help sometimes and complete help always) was rated for several areas of activities of daily living (ADL). In the sample of impaired adults 30% of all patients were in need of partial to full help at all times in (nearly) all areas of daily living (bathing, dressing, appearance, feeding, etc). In the sample of impaired children, ADL was computed for children older than six (younger children normally need help in ADL). In this sample, the majority of children also needed partial to full help some of the time in all areas of daily living.

CAREGIVING VARIABLES

For the adult sample, the caregiving duration was less than one year for 29 (16%) caregivers, one to three years for 51 (28%) caregivers, four to nine years for 60 (33%), ten to twenty years for 33 (18%) and more than twenty years for eight (5%) caregivers. About half of the patients needed 24-hour care, 13% needed some additional care throughout the day, 19% needed between two to six hours care per day, and only 18% needed less than 2 to 6 hours of care. Thirty-seven percent of the caregivers felt that the patient's health status was growing worse, 30% considered it stable, 26% perceived ups and downs, and 7% felt that the patient's health was improving.

As for the population of children, the care giving duration was less than one year for 4 (4.3%) caregivers, one to two years for 9 (9.8%), two to four years for 14 (15.2%), five to ten years for 32 (34.8%) and ten and more years for 33 (35.9%). About 16% of the child population needed care due to their disability day and night, and 33% needed care all day (beyond what is required by regular care for a child). When asked about the child's condition, 13% of the caregivers reported that the situation was worsening, 44% perceived no change in the situation, and 34% thought the situation was improving. The number of elderly patients with only *physical* impairment was twice as large as in the children's sample. The number of persons with mental problems only was more in the child than in the adult sample. The caregiving duration was longer for more caregivers in the child sample than in the aging sample while the number of hours of care per day was greater for the population of impaired adults and elderly.

FINDINGS AND DISCUSSION

In any discussion of families' attitudes towards institutional care for their family members, we must be clear in distinguishing at which point of time along the caregiving trajectory respondents were questioned. All of our caregivers had, by virtue of accepting the responsibility of homecare, rejected the possibility of institutionalization at the onset of illness.

There is no question that both caregivers of the aged, as well as caregivers of children, do face and make this choice over and over. Old people are institutionalized after hospitalization for a stroke or fracture; multiple handicapped or retarded children are institutionalized with diagnosis often following birth. In our samples, all the families had chosen homecare and were involved in its daily reality—74% of the persons caring for adults and 85% of the persons caring for children had been giving care for at least two years.

We are, in fact, addressing the question of how caregivers already under a usually heavy burden for a prolonged period of time view institutionalization and which variables seem to encourage or discourage continuing homecare. The dilemma facing caregivers is eloquently expressed by one family member:

> But he is Levison! How can a man such as Levison be in an institution? I owe it to myself, as his wife, to care for him; I owe it to him, even if it is terrible. But would it be easier if he were in an institution? I would be there all day; my conscience wouldn't give me a minute's peace. As long as possible, I must, I must continue.

Another caregiver comments: "As long as she recognizes me, as long as it makes a difference for her, she will stay in her home!" The mother of a nine-year-old retarded boy states: "Now he is restless; we hardly have a quiet minute, but we want and need him close. Still, he will grow up; what shall we do if he becomes violent and we are old?"

For many caregivers, the mere fact that the impaired person (adult or child) was present answered some basic psychological need (e.g., love, being needed, meaning in life). But the overriding sense of these caregivers, faced with the alternative of institutionalization while under a heavy caregiving burden, was that of a double bind:

> I am damned if I continue homecare; I am damned if I don't. I have already accepted my fate. So, I don't go out; so, I can't hear a concert; so, my back hurts, and I am too tired and exhausted to cry; but how could I have a joyful minute; how could I have a peaceful night's sleep, knowing I "deserted" him in an institution?

We shall present our findings according to the study questions:

1. What are the caregivers' feelings regarding the continuation of homecare?
2. What are the caregivers' attitudes toward institutionalization?
3. Are the caregivers' feelings regarding continuation of homecare and their attitudes toward institutionalization similar or different in child versus aged caring?
4. Are feelings toward continuation of homecare and attitudes toward institutionalization of child and aged carers related to:
    (4.1) Demographic variables?
    (4.2) Illness variables?
    (4.3) Caregiving variables?
    (4.4) Caregiving resources?
    (4.5) The caregivers' perception of the caregiving burden (cost)?
    (4.6) The caregivers' quality of relationship to the patient?
    (4.7) The caregivers' tolerance and management ability of patient symptoms and behaviors?

1. Caregivers were asked to respond to a closed question describing their feelings toward continued homecare for their patients on a five point scale. Table 1 shows that the large majority of both populations (childcare 87%, adult carers 77.3%) receive gratification from homecare. Only 9.7% of the childcarers and 5.6% of the aged carers feel subjected to homecare out of "no choice."

2. Caregivers were asked to respond to a closed question describing their attitude towards institutionalization of their patient on a five point scale. Table 2 shows that the large majority of both populations (childcarers, 82.6%; caretakers for adults, 75.7%) reject institutionalization as a viable option. Only few want to place their patient in an institution (childcarers 10.9%; caretakers for adults 11.6%).

3. In contrast to what might be expected from social stereotypes, there is no difference between childcarers and aged carers as to their feelings toward homecare and their attitude

TABLE 1

CAREGIVER FEELING TOWARD CONTINUED HOMECARE

Feeling Toward Continued Homecare	Childcarers		Carers for Adults	
	N	%	N	%
The presence of the patient at home gives great emotional gratification.	23	25.0	54	29.8
Caring for the patient is a duty which also gives gratification.	57	62.0	86	47.5
Caring for the patient is a moral duty only	3	3.3	23	12.7
Care is continued out of the feeling of "no other choice"	4	4.3	7	3.9
Continued care at home is unbearable.	5	5.4	3	1.7
Blank	0	0	8	4.4
Total	92	100.0	181	100.0

TABLE 2

CAREGIVER ATTITUDE TOWARD INSTITUTIONALIZATION

Attitude Toward Institutionalization	Childcarers		Carers for Adults	
	N	%	N	%
Unwilling to consider institution- alization even for the future.	64	69.6	103	56.9
Willing to consider institution- alization as a last resort.	12	13.0	34	18.8
Willing to consider institution- alization under certain circumstances (not for now).	6	6.5	15	8.3
Willing to place the patient in an institution, but taking no steps.	2	2.2	9	5.0
In process of institutionalization.	8	8.7	12	6.6
Blank	0	0	8	4.4
Total	92	100.0	181	100.0

towards institutionalization, once these families have opted for homecare in the past. There is no question that our research describes "survivors" who, in the face of tremendous hardship, wish to continue homecare. The ability of caregivers to obtain emotional gratification from caregiving seems to be the crucial variable influencing the future of homecare. The correlations of feelings toward continued homecare and attitudes toward institutionalization were statistically significant in both populations (childcarers $r = .48$, $p < .001$; adult carers $r = .51$, $p < .001$). The moment homecare is perceived only as a duty, institutionalization becomes a viable option.

Demographic Variables and Continuation of Care (Caregiver Feelings Toward Continued Homecare and Caregiver Attitudes Toward Institutionalization)

Demographic variables made close to no difference in caretakers of adults, and some difference in childcarers regarding the continuation of care.

Carers for Adults

The only variable making a slight difference for caretakers of adults was the patient's sex. Caregivers tended to perceive caring for a male as more of an obligation ($r = .14$, $p < .03$). It seems that caregivers of men (usually spouses or daughters) tend to continue homecare even when they do not feel satisfaction from caregiving and consider it only a duty. Even when demographic differences are accounted for, women are over-represented in the institutionalized population.

Caregivers' attitudes toward institutionalization were not influenced by the patient's sex. Patient's age, country of origin, and level of education also made no significant difference regarding continuation of care. We know from the literature (Kastenbaum, 1983; Kop, 1980) that the likelihood of institutionalization increases greatly with age, mainly because of dwindling resources. However, by virtue of the sample selection method (the fact that people were actually able to provide care), we interviewed only families where at least minimum caregiving resources were available.

An unexpected finding in our research is that kinship (i.e.

the relationship of caregiver to the patient) does not make a difference in continuation of care.

Johnson (1983) in a study of family supports of 167 post-hospitalized individuals over age 65 reports that the spouse had a critical role in preventing institutionalization. Also, in our sample, 72.3% of those who were actually providing homecare were spouses, but they were not more likely than children to feel positively about care or reject institutionalization.

Caregivers' sex, age, country of origin, level of education, employment status, economic resources, and socio-economic status were not significantly related to continuation of homecare. The fact that socio-economic status did not make a difference does indicate that at least basic economic needs, which are a precondition to homecare, were covered (i.e., housing, health care, and minimal income).

The fact that the level of religious observance (from atheist to orthodox) and country of origin did not make a statistically significant difference in regard to institutionalization refutes widespread stereotypes of religious rather than non-religious people and "Orientals" rather than "Europeans" being willing and able to provide unconditional long-term care to their aged.

Child Carers

For the childcarers, the sex of the child, the number of siblings, the mother's level of education, the family's economic resources, and socio-economic status all made some difference in regard to continuation of homecare (feelings and attitudes of mothers).

From Table 3, we see that boys (boys = 0, girls = 1) have a better chance for continued homecare and that lower education, more children, and less economic resources increase the likelihood of institutionalization.

These findings are congruent with the literature (Stone, 1967; Chigier, 1969; Vidan, 1980). There is no question that low socio-economic status, many young children, and the disadvantage of low education, combined, spell scarce family resources toward shouldering the heavy burden of continued homecare.

Also, childcarers' country of origin and level of religious

TABLE 3

CHILDCARERS AND CONTINUATION OF HOMECARE   (N=92)

Demographic Variables	Feelings Toward Continued Homecare	Attitudes Toward Institutionalization
Child sex	r=.23, p<.01	r=.17, p<.04
Number of siblings	N.S.	r=.20 p<.02
Mother's educational level	N.S.	r=-.18 p<.03
Economic resources	r=.17, p<.04	r=.18, p<.04
SES	N.S.	r=-.16 p<.05

observance made no difference in the families' willingness and ability to continue homecare.

There were no statistically significant correlations between the child's age, the mother's age, employment status, and the mother's attitudes towards the continuation of homecare. The fact that the child's age made no difference is not congruent with the literature, where Stone (1967) and Chigier (1969) report that parents of older children are more likely to consider institutionalization.

Illness Variables and Continuation of Homecare

For both children and adults the kind of impairment made a statistically significant difference in regard to the caregiver's feelings toward continuation of homecare. The kind of impairment made no statistically significant difference in caregivers' attitudes toward institutionalization. For the subsample of families with impaired adults, cross-tabulation analysis shows that there is least emotional satisfaction in caring for mentally impaired persons and most satisfaction in the care of those who have only physical impairment ($x^2 =$ 18.527, sig. 001). For the subsample of families with impaired children, analysis of variance demonstrates that there is least emotional satisfaction in the care of mentally impaired children. (See Table 4.)

ADL functioning or degree of dependence made no difference in either adults or children in regard to the continuation of homecare. Klusmann et al. (1981) in their longitudinal

TABLE 4

CHILDGIVERS' FEELINGS TOWARD CONTINUED HOMECARE
AND KIND OF IMPAIRMENT

Source	DF	SS	MS	F
Kind of impairment	3	3.710	1.23	3.63
Error	88	29.975	.341	
Total	91	33.685		

P<.016

study of homecare, shed light on the question of the relation-ship between level of the patient's dependency and the family's attitudes toward institutionalization. They also found no difference in the above when analyzing the answers of families providing homecare. But when they looked at which old people had been institutionalized after 15 months, they did find that the degree of dependency made a statistically significant difference. Their explanation highlights the fact that there is a self-selection element in caregivers continuing homecare, despite severe functional impairment.

For the 145 adult patients who had one of the seven fol-lowing illnesses as their first diagnosis: heart disease, Parkin-son's disease, diabetes, bone or joint diseases, cancer, cere-brovascular accident, and dementia, there was no statistically significant difference in their caregivers' attitude toward con-tinued homecare.

Caregiving Variables and Continuation of Homecare

Caregiving duration and intensity of care (number of hours per day) made no difference in either subsample in regard to continuation of homecare. However, the caregiver's percep-tion of the illness trajectory was statistically significant in in-fluencing feelings toward continued homecare and attitudes towards institutionalization. Whenever caretakers for adults thought the situation would deteriorate, rather than remain stable, fluctuate or improve, they were more likely to con-sider institutionalization. ($r = -.22, p < .001$).

Also, the childcarers were influenced by their perception of the trajectory. There is a statistically significant correlation between the mother's perception of improvement versus deterioration and their attitudes toward continuation of homecare. The more they considered the situation to deteriorate, the more they felt bound to the care out of "no choice" or duty only ($r = .21, p < .02$) and the more they were willing to consider institutionalization ($r = .33, p < .001$).

Caregiving Resources and Continuation of Homecare

Caregivers' Physical and Mental Health

For families with impaired adults caregivers' overall assessment of their own physical health, as well as their functional capacity (IADL) made no difference in regard to continuation of care. But, whenever caretakers regarded caregiving to negatively affect their physical health, they tended to view institutionalization more favourably ($r = .23, p < .001$).

Mothers of impaired children who reported more physical symptoms related to caregiving also tended to view institutionalization as an option ($r = .26, p < .006$).

Caregivers were asked how frequently they experienced several emotional states. The frequency of their occurrence correlated with attitudes toward continuing homecare. The findings in Table 5 illustrate how the caregiver's physical and mental health affect continuation of homecare for both impaired adults and children.

Family and Social Resources

Caregivers were asked to rate their overall social resources and those of their patients; their ability to receive and enjoy both practical and emotional support; and the amount of involvement of family and others in the care. Caretakers were also asked whether they felt that their effort was appreciated by other people.

As Table 6 shows, the caregiver's sense of satisfaction from caring versus her/his feeling of being trapped is decisively influenced by the social support available. Interestingly enough, the

TABLE 5

EMOTIONAL STATES AND CONTINUED HOMECARE

Emotional State	Feelings Toward Continued Homecare		Attitudes Toward Institutionalization	
	Child Carers	Aged Carers	Child Carers	Aged Carers
Depression	r=.32 p<.001	r=.36 p<.001	r=.40 p<.001	r=.20 p<.01
Aggression	r=.21 p<.03	N.S.	r=.32 p<.004	N.S.
Anxiety	N.S.	N.S.	N.S.	r=.15 p<.05
Restlessness	N.S.	–	N.S.	–
Listlessness	N.S.	–	N.S.	–
Tension	r=.19 p<.03	r=.21 p<.01	r=.22 p<.02	N.S.

TABLE 6

FAMILY AND SOCIAL RESOURCES

Family and Social Resources	Feelings Toward Continued Homecare		Attitudes Toward Institutionalization	
	Child Carers	Carers for Adults	Child Carers	Carers for Adults
Overal social resources – patient	r=.41 p<.001	r=.27 p<.001	r=.26 p<.005	N.S.
Overall social resources – caregiver	N.S.	r=.20 p<.003	N.S.	N.S.
Ability to receive/enjoy practical support	r=.24 p<.008	r=.21 p<.001	N.S.	N.S.
Ability to receive/enjoy emotional support	r=.02 p<.02	r=.26 p<.001	N.S.	N.S.
Degree of involvement of family/ others	N.S.	N.S.	N.S.	N.S.
Degree of involvement of children	N.S.	r=.14 p<.03	N.S.	N.S.
Appreciation of others	–	r=.29 p<.001	–	r=.19 p<.004

strongest correlation relates to how caregivers perceive the patients' social resources, rather than their own. The fewer the patient's resources, the more continued care was thought of as a duty or a "no alternative" option. We wonder whether this finding might be explained by one or more of the following factors:

1. Patients with fewer social resources are "objectively" less desirable (e.g., repugnant);
2. The fewer the patient's social resources, the more the primary caregiver is the sole substitute for companionship, adding to the caregiving burden;
3. Low social desirability also affects the primary relationship.

The less mothers were able to recruit and enjoy support, the less they were able to gain emotional satisfaction from caregiving.

Caretakers for adults felt better about continuation of homecare whenever there were more overall social resources, more involvement of their children, more appreciation of their efforts from others, and when they were able to recruit and enjoy support.

While for the child carers the only variable influencing attitudes toward institutionalization was the child's social resources: the less resources, the higher the tendency toward institutionalization. Perceived appreciation of others was the only variable which made a difference for caretakers of adults. The more caregivers felt their efforts were appreciated by others, the less they tended toward institutionalization. The fact that social support makes the overriding difference in the caregiver's feelings about homecare, and *not* in their willingness to institutionalize, underlines the fact that we are reporting about a population of "survivors."

These findings are congruent with the literature on social support which indicates that social support functions as a moderating variable that facilitates coping with stressful situations. Social support also provides a protective function, easing the physiological and psychological consequences of chronic strain (Cassel, 1976; Cobb, 1976; Norbeck, 1981).

Professional Involvement

This study demonstrates the inadequacy of community long-term care. There is a severe imbalance between the severity of conditions and professional help available. Mothers as a whole perceived the involvement of physicians, nurses, social workers, and others to be minimal, which made it impossible to analyze the effect of professional involvement upon continuation of homecare. Compared to the needs of the adult population, the amount of professional involvement was also inadequate. Nevertheless, for the aged population, there was some relationship between the continuation of homecare and amount of professional involvement. (See Table 7)

Whenever there was more physician involvement, families were less likely to tend toward institutionalization and felt caregiving less of a "no choice" alternative. It is not clear whether physicians actually "made the difference," or whether more "positive" families were more likely to receive medical attention. Since an important part of the home care team's duties is the facilitation of institutionalization, it is not surprising that more contact with the team is related to more positive

TABLE 7

IMPACT OF PROFESSIONAL RESOURCES ON CONTINUATION

OF HOMECARE FOR CAREGIVERS OF ADULTS

Professional Involvement	Feelings Toward Continuation of Homecare	Attitudes Toward Institutionalization
Physician	$r=-.12$ $p < .04$	$r=-.20$ $p < .003$
Nurse	N.S.	N.S.
Home Care Team	N.S.	$r=.15$ $p < .02$
Social Work	N.S.	N.S.
Physiotherapy	N.S.	$r=-.12$ $p < .05$
Occupational Therapy	N.S.	N.S.

attitudes about institutionalization among caregivers. A major indication for receiving physiotherapy is rehabilitation potential. This means that patients who are "better off" to begin with (i.e., without mental impairment and with less general decline) are more likely to receive physiotherapy. For these patients, there is less reason to consider institutionalization. From a social and health care policy standpoint, the above findings raise serious questions.

Impact of Caregiving Cost Upon Continuation of Homecare

The burden (or cost) of caretaking is described in the literature as a crucial variable influencing homecare (Isaacs et al., 1972; Archbold, 1982; Holt, 1975; Farber, 1960).

Table 8 demonstrates the relationships between an overall measure of cost, the ten areas of the caregivers' lives where perceived impact of caregiving cost was measured, and attitudes toward continuation of homecare.

Impact of Caretaking on Families with Impaired Children

Table 8 shows that the more mothers felt their physical health, sense of security, and their relationship to the child to be influenced negatively by caregiving, the more they tended to perceive continued homecare as a duty or "no choice" situation. Perceived negative impact upon physical health, security, as well as sleep and rest, correlated with mothers' increased tendency toward institutionalization. The relationship between negative impact of caregiving on caretaker's health and the tendency to institutionalize is documented in the literature (Vidan, 1980; Holt, 1975). In her study of 40 Israeli families who cared for retarded children at home and 48 families who were in the process of institutionalizing their retarded child, Vidan (1980) reported that the latter group perceived more stress and disruption in different life areas than the former. Stone (1967) and Farber (1960a) found that whenever caregiving influenced family relationships negatively, families were more likely to place a retarded child in an institution. This last finding was not born out by our sample.

TABLE 8

THE IMPACT OF PERCEIVED COST AND CONTINUATION OF
HOMECARE FOR CARETAKERS OF IMPAIRED CHILDREN AND ADULTS

Cost	Feelings Toward Continuation of Homecare		Attitudes Toward Institutionalization	
	Child Carers	Carers for Adults	Child Carers	Carers for Adults
Cost Index (overall measure)	N.S.	r=.25 p<.001	N.S.	r=.26 p<.001
Physical Health	r=.18 p<.04	N.S.	r=.17 p<.05	r=.23 p<.001
Mental health	N.S.	N.S.	N.S.	N.S.
Ability to go out	N.S	r=.27 p<.001	N.S.	N.S
Privacy	N.S.	r=.14 p<.03	N.S.	r=.21 p<.002
Sleep and rest	N.S.	r=.27 p<.001	r=.27 p<.005	N.S.
Employment	N.S.	N.S.	N.S.	N.S.
Security	r=.22 p<.02	N.S.	r=.27 p<.004	N.S.
Family relationships	N.S.	r=.22 p<.002	N.S.	r=.21 p<.002
Social relationships	N.S	N.S.	N.S.	N.S.
Relationship with patient	r=.23 p<.015	r=.38 p<.001	N.S.	r=.28 p<.001

Impact of Caregiving on Families with Impaired Adult

In contrast to the childcarers, the overall measure of cost did make a difference for caretakers of adults. The higher the cost, the more caregivers considered homecare out of duty or "no choice" only, and the more institutionalization seemed a viable option. A perceived negative impact of caring upon "ability to go out," privacy and family relationships correlated with negative feelings toward continued homecare. A perceived negative impact of caring upon physical health, privacy, and family relationships correlated with a tendency to consider institutionalization. Whenever caretakers perceived caregiving to have a negative impact upon their relationship to the patient, the probability of continued homecare declined.

Patient-Caregiver Relationship and Continuation of Homecare

The patient-caregiver relationship, defined as mutuality, was identified as the crucial variable determining caregivers' tendency to continue homecare versus considering institutionalization for impaired adults (Hirschfeld, 1983). In our present study, several items were aimed at gaining evidence on the interdependency of the caregiving relationship (Table 9).

All four relationship variables correlated significantly with carers' feelings toward continued homecare for impaired adults. The less appreciation from the patient, the more gratitude was absent; the more the caregivers perceived caregiving to negatively influence their relationship to the patient, and the greater the relief when imagining the loss of the patient; the more carers viewed continued homecare as an obligation or "no choice" situation, and the more willing they were to consider institution-

TABLE   9

PATIENT–CAREGIVER RELATIONSHIP AND

CONTINUATION OF HOMECARE

Patient–Caregiver Relationship	Feelings Toward Continuation of Homecare		Attitude Towards Institutionalization	
	Child Carers	Aged Carers	Child Carers	Aged Carers
Appreciation from patient	N.S.	r=.34 p<.001	N.S.	r=.30 p<.001
Quality of caregiver– patient relationship	r=.23 p<.01	r=.38 p<.001	N.S.	r=.28 p<.001
Caregiver imagining loss of patient	–	r=.31 p<.001	–	r=.30 p<.001
Absence of patient gratitude	r=.24 p<.01	r=.38 p<.001	r=.46 p<.001	r=.25 p<.001

alization of the impaired adult. Mothers felt more negatively toward continued homecare whenever they perceived the quality of their relationship to be negatively influenced by caregiving and whenever the child showed no gratitude. It is interesting that lack of gratitude is the only relationship item influencing mothers to consider institutionalization.

This study highlights the importance of caregiver-patient interrelationship variables, not only in caregiving for adults and aged, but also for those caring for children. This is a crucial caregiving aspect which, to the best of our knowledge, have not yet been reported in the literature. Nevertheless, there seem to be differences for both populations. While adults are expected to appreciate the efforts of their caregivers, less is expected of children in this area. While the perceived negative impact of caregiving upon the relationship influences the attitudes of caretakers of adults to consider institutionalization, this factor is not sufficient to make a difference in mothers' tendencies to institutionalize their handicapped child.

Caregivers' Tolerance of and Ability to Manage Patients' Symptoms/Behaviors and Continuation of Homecare

This section deals with the impact of symptom-tolerance and management upon continuation of homecare (Table 10).

A correlation between the symptom-tolerance and management index and the caregivers' feelings toward continuation of homecare was statistically significant for both populations (childcarers: $r = .46$ $p < .001$; carers of adults: $r = .38$, $p < .001$). Caretakers felt more positive toward continued homecare whenever they were able to tolerate and manage symptoms better.

While the same index correlated significantly with the childcarers' attitudes toward institutionalization ($r = .49$, $p < .001$), less symptom-tolerance and management ability did not influence attitudes about institutionalization for caretakers of impaired adults.

In addition to the overall index, the following describes how tolerance and management ability of various symptoms/behaviors relate to continued homecare. Caretakers were asked whether each of the symptoms/behaviors existed and, when present, if caretakers considered them (1) "not a problem", (2) "a manageable problem", (3) "a problem managed with difficulty" and (4) or "an intolerable problem". Results are presented in Table 11.

While incontinence and difficulties with verbal interaction were symptoms frequently faced by childcarers, falls and problems with hearing, vision and sleep were more frequent problems confronting caretakers for adults. While for mothers, the inability to tolerate and manage all symptoms, except hearing and vision were positively correlated with negative feelings toward homecare, for caretakers of adults, only the inability to tolerate and manage fecal incontinence, speech and hearing impairment, and confusion were correlated with negative feelings toward continued homecare. While for childcarers, the inability to tolerate and manage all symptoms (except hearing and vision impairment) was positively correlated with the growing willingness to place a child in an institution, for carers of adults, only the inability to tolerate and manage confusional states increased the likelihood of placement. The tolerance of other symptoms was not statistically significant in explaining placement attitudes.

While dangerous behaviors, nagging, restlessness, and lack of cooperation had to be faced more frequently by childcarers; aggression, apathy, depression, and crying were behaviors carers of adults had to deal with more frequently (see Table 11). Inability to tolerate and manage most of these behaviors was positively correlated with negative feelings toward continued homecare for both groups of caregivers. The inability of mothers to tolerate/manage dangerous and aggressive behaviors, restlessness, apathy, depression, and crying was positively correlated with a tendency to institutionalize. In the literature (Holt, 1975; Maney et al., 1964), restlessness, aggressive behaviors, and other behavioral disturbances are mentioned as key factors leading to placement of a retarded child. For caretakers of adults, only argumentative, uncooperative, and apathetic behaviors contributed to the willingness to consider institutionalization.

SUMMARY OF FINDINGS

Our research described survivors who in the face of tremendous hardship wish to continue homecare to their severely impaired children and adult relatives. In contrast to

TABLE 10

CAREGIVERS' TOLERANCE AND MANAGEMENT ABILITY OF SYMPTOMS AND CONTINUED HOMECARE

SYMPTOMS	% of Patients with Symptoms		Feelings Toward Continued Homecare		Attitudes Toward Institutionalization	
	Child	Aged	Child Carers	Aged Carers	Child Carers	Aged Carers
Urinary incontinence	56.5	42.5	r=.31 p<.001	N.S.	r=.26 p<.005	N.S.
Fecal incontinence	5.7	28.7	r=.24 p<.01	r=.15 p<.02	r=.33 p<.001	N.S.
Falls and instability	56.5	69.6	r=.27 p<.004	N.S.	r=.30 p<.001	N.S.
Difficulty under-standing language	46.7	21.5	r=.20 p<.02	N.S.	r=.31 p<.001	N.S.
Speech Impairment	66.3	33.7	r=.26 p<.005	r=.18 p<.006	r=.29 p<.002	N.S.
Hearing impairment	12.0	30.4	N.S.	r=.29 p<.001	N.S.	N.S.
Vision impairment	27.2	42.0	N.S.	N.S.	N.S.	N.S.
Confusion	26.1	27.1	r=.37 p<.001	r=.24 p<.001	r=.28 p<.003	r=.29 p<.006
Sleep disturbance	43.5	64.1	r=.32 p<.001	N.S.	r=.51 p<.001	N.S.

TABLE 11

CAREGIVERS' TOLERANCE AND MANAGEMENT OF BEHAVIORS AND CONTINUED HOMECARE

BEHAVIORS	% of Patients with Behavior		Feeling Toward Continued Homecare		Attitudes Toward Institutionalization	
	Child	Aged	Child Carers	Aged Carers	Child Carers	Aged Carers
Dangerous Behavior	32.6	6.1	$r=.25$ $p<.007$	$r=.14$ p .03	$r=.36$ $p<.001$	N.S.
Violent and aggressive	32.6	71.3	$r=.37$ $p<.001$	N.S.	$r=.18$ $p<.03$	N.S.
Getting lost	18.5	4.4	N.S.	N.S.	N.S.	N.S.
Nagging	64.1	42.5	$r=.20$ $p<.02$	$r=.27$ $p<.001$	N.S.	N.S.
Argumentative	—	28.2	—	$r=.32$ $p<.001$	—	$r=.26$ $p<.001$
Restless	52.2	23.8	$r=.44$ $p<.001$	$r=.22$ $p<.002$	$r=.27$ $p<.004$	N.S.
Uncooperative	46.7	28.2	$r=.41$ $p<.001$	$r=.43$ $p<.001$	N.S.	$r=.22$ $p<.001$
Apathetic	29.1	37.2	$r=.26$ $p<.006$	$r=.31$ $p<.001$	$r=.33$ $p<.001$	$r=.15$ $p<.02$
Unwilling to get out of bed	17.4	24.9	N.S.	$r=.17$ $p<.009$	N.S.	N.S.
Depressed/crying	28.0	58.6	N.S.	$r=.15$ $p<.025$	$r=.23$ $p<.01$	N.S.

what might be expected from social stereotypes there is little difference betweeen childcarers and caregivers to elderly adults in their attitudes toward continuation of home-care. Several major findings arise from this study:

1. The majority of both caregiver populations receive gratification from their ability to care for their patient at home.
2. The variation of caregivers' feelings toward continued homecare was related to several variables. Negative feelings toward continued homecare correspond with:
   a. the patients' mental impairment rather than physical impairment
   b. the perception of a deteriorating illness trajectory
   c. the occurrence of depression, aggression and tension in the caregivers
   d. the absence of sufficient social support
   e. the absence of professional homecare services
3. The majority of caregivers to both populations rejected institutionalization as a viable option.
4. The variation of caregivers' attitudes towards institutionalization was also related to several variables. Caregivers who were willing to consider institutionalization as a potential alternative to homecare were:
   a. In the sample of child carers those mothers who have a number of small children, who had a lower level of formal education and less economic resources. Demographic variables made no difference for the caregivers to adults;
   b. in both sub-samples those caregivers who perceived their patient to deteriorate;
   c. in both sub-samples those caregivers who felt that their physical health was negatively effected by caregiving;
   d. in both sub-samples those who considered themselves depressed and anxious.
5. The way caregivers perceived their caregiving responsibilities to effect their own lives influenced both their feelings toward continuation of home care, as well as attitudes toward institutionalization. A perceived negative effect upon the caregivers' physical health, sleep

and rest, privacy and sense of security was related to a growing sense of home care as an unbearable situation and a willingness to consider institutionalization.

6. The ability of caregivers to tolerate and manage symptoms and behaviors of their patients made a significant difference in their feelings toward continued homecare and their attitudes toward institutionalization. Less ability to tolerate/manage symptoms had greater weight in the child carer sample than in the carers of aged. In addition continuation of homecare for child carers was influenced by their ability to tolerate/manage dangerous/violent/aggressive behaviors, while for caregivers of the aged continued home care was more influenced by apathetic/uncooperative and argumentative behaviors.

7. The quality of the caregiver-patient relationship and the perceived gratitude of patients in both populations were crucial for a positive outlook toward continuation of home care.

The findings of our research seem to highlight a phenomenon of great importance to health care providers. While the demographic variables, which we are unable to influence, made close to no difference in families' attitudes toward home care versus institutionalization, several elements as the burden of caregiving, the management ability of a caregiver and the quality of the patient-caregiver relationship made significant differences. All of these elements are amenable to change.

Implications for Services

Our findings indicate that services must be aimed toward three major goals:

1. the decrease of negative impact upon the caregivers' life
2. the increase of the caregiver's tolerance and management ability of patient symptoms and behaviors and
3. the creation of circumstances, which potentially enhance the quality of the caregiver-patient relationship.

An important premise for creating adequate services is the

realization that home care and institutional services are neither opposed to one another, nor mutually exclusive. Care of such patients asks for shared responsibility of both families and professional service providers. Services can be alternately provided in the home, the community or the institution. Health care policy must plan these services as complimentary and multidirectional in order to answer the complex and ever changing needs.

Services have two main purposes. The first purpose lies in helping the family, in particular the prime caregiver to cope with home care. The second purpose is to provide temporary relief of caregiving responsibilities and at times support ultimate institutionalization. Multi-disciplinary home care teams must provide the following services geared toward primary, secondary and tertiary prevention and care for both the patient and the family: comprehensive nursing care addressing the physical, cognitive, emotional, social and environmental needs, physiotherapy, occupational therapy, social work and continued medical monitoring. Overall responsibility for the care of a family remains with the nurse. Direct care provision, as well as patient and family teaching are needed from all members of the team.

Family caregivers must be recognized as a population "at risk" and special attention should be paid to their potential stress related diseases as high blood pressure, tension headaches, obesity, cardiovascular problems, anxiety states and depression.

Following we shall focus upon the role of the nurse in caring for these families of children and aged alike: Caregivers need guidance in developing coping strategies to reduce the negative impact of the caregiving situation on the different aspects of their lives. Among other issues: how caregiving can be shared more effectively; how time and other resources can be best divided among all family members; how to assess and use the strength of a family's social network; it is of great importance to encourage and "legitimize" the prime caregiver in answering her/his own needs for privacy, some pleasurable activities, rest etc. Practical guidance must be directed toward improving management strategies as, e.g., lifting a patient, handling restless or aggressive behavior or modifying the physical environment. There is a need for a non-judgmental listener helping the caregiver to work through her/his emotional reactions to the partial loss of the impaired person. The entire family needs counseling toward finding a modus vivendi where each member can contribute and receive some support, despite the objective hardships.

For temporarily relieving caregivers, a wide array of services are needed: (1) a free or low-cost sitter service; (2) low-cost comprehensive day care services ready to accommodate individuals who are both mentally and physically impaired (including the incontinent individual and the person with a tendency to wander or to aggressive behavior). Day care must include transportation services and be available for at least two full days per week to be effective in relieving strain; (3) respite services enabling the caregiver to take a "vacation." Live-in non-professional low-cost assistance would ideally leave the senile brain-diseased person, or the retarded child in his/her accustomed environment (and prevent disrupting his/her precarious balance by a residential move), while enabling the caregiver to get some rest and replenish energies. Most family members in this study desperately wanted to visit relatives or friends, or take a trip—"just for some time off." Another alternative to live-in respite services would be low cost beds in long-term care institutions allocated to short-term care with the explicit objective of granting the caregivers temporary relief.

While in Israel the need for aged-respite services is at least, theoretically accepted, the need for child-respite services has yet to enter public consciousness. The actual availability of respite care for both population groups is, at present, close to nil. Whenever the above alternatives are not effective or desired by the caregiver to reduce the family's tension, these families deserve the prerogative of choice with appropriate institutions providing good nursing care. Such institutions must be available and financially accessible to be a possible alternative to home care. No one should be made to feel guilty for their "failure" to keep a person with senile brain disease, or an autistic child, at home. Many caregivers in the study felt guilty whenever considering institutionalization as a possible alternative. Whenever a family does decide to institutionalize an impaired person, a professional placement service is needed to assist the families in placing their relative in an institution most suitable to the individual's needs and the family's needs. Institutional placement may at times be in the best interest of the patient.

Education of health care personnel is an extremely important area, but beyond the scope of this article.

Implications for Further Research

This study suggested the need for research in major areas:

1. methodological research to establish the armamentaria necessary to measure family impact of home care versus institutionalization;
2. added knowledge on the development of family coping over time in relation to the length of the caregiving situation, the kind of impairment, and the point on the individual and family life cycle;
3. development and evaluation of effective nursing interventions for dependent populations and their families;
4. evaluation program research in regard to services for families living with disease;
5. cross-cultural research on families in caregiving situations.

REFERENCES

Archbold, P.G. (1982). An analysis of parentcaring by women. *Home Health Care Services Quarterly, 3*(2), 5–25.

Cassel, J. (1976). The contribution of social environment to host resistance. *American Journal of Epidemiology, 104*, 107–123.

Chigier, E. (1969). *Mongolism in Tel Aviv.* Jerusalem: Research project B SS-CD-IS-6, Medical Ecology Department, Hebrew University Medical School.

Coll, S. (1976). Social support as a moderator of life stress. *Psychosomatic Medicine, 38*, 300-314.

Farber, B. (1960). Perception of crisis and related variables in the impact of a retarded child on the mother. *Journal of Health and Human Behavior, 1*, 108–118.

Hirschfeld, M. (1978). Families living with senile brain disease. Doctoral dissertation. University of California, San Francisco. University Microfilms No. 295400.

Hirschfeld, M. (1983). Homecare versus institutionalization: family caregiving and senile brain disease. *International Journal of Nursing Studies, 20*(1), 23–32.

Holt, K.S. (1975). Home care of severely retarded children. In J.J. Dempsey (Ed.), *Community Services for Retarded Children* (pp. 65–78). Baltimore: University Park Press.

Isaacs, B., Livingstone, M., Neville, I. (1972). *Survival of the unfittest.* London: Routledge and Kegan Paul.

Israel National Report to the U.N. World Assembly on Aging. (1982). *Aging in Israel*. Jerusalem, Israel: Monograph submitted to the Ministry of Labor and Social Affairs and to the Ministry of Foreign Affairs.

Johnson, C.L. (1983). Dyadic family relations and social support. *Gerontologist*, *23*(4), 377–383.

Kastenbaum, R. (1983). The 4% Fallacy: R.I.P. *International Journal of Aging and Human Development*. *17*(1), 71–74.

Klusmann, D., Bruder, J., Lanter, H., and Luders, I. (1981). *Beziehungen zwischen patienten und ihren familienangchönigen bei chronischen erkrankungen des höheren lebensalters*. Hamburg: Bericht an die Deutsche Forschungsgemeinschaft Teilprojekt A 16, Sonderforsch ungsbereich 115.

Kop, Y. (1980). *Changes in the age structure and their implication for demand for public services*. Jerusalem: Joint (JDC) Brookdale Institute of Gerontology and Adult Human Behavior, D-64-80.

Krulik, T. (1978). Loneliness in school age children living with chronic life threatening illness. Doctoral dissertation. University of California, San Francisco. University Microfilm No. CZN79–05548.

Krulik, T., and Hirschfeld, M. (1984). Family Caregiving to Severe Chronically Ill Children and Aged. Research Monograph. Tel Aviv: Tel Aviv University.

Maney, A.C., Pace, R., Morrison, D.F. (1964). A factor Analytic Study of the need for Institutionalization. *American Journal of Mental Deficiency*, *69*, 372–384.

Norbeck, J. (1981). Social support–A model for clinical research and application. *Advances in Nursing Science*, *3*, 43–59.

Stone, N.D. (1967). Family factors in willingness to place the mongoloid child. *American Journal of Mental Deficiency*, *72*(1), 16–20.

Vidan, N. (1980). Coping of families with a retarded child. Israel: University of Haifa, unpublished masters thesis.

The United States:
Long-Term Care and Federal Policy

Carroll L. Estes, PhD

ABSTRACT. Examines the need for uniform national policy for the provision of long-term care (LTC) services at an affordable price with access for all in need; points up the relationship between LTC issues and acute care policy; outlines seven basic principles for a comprehensive LTC system; lists problems to be solved and proposes alternative solutions for issues of chronicity, access, and cost control; and urges long-range comprehensive policy reform for health care delivery and financing.

The dream of a national system of long-term care services at an affordable price with access for those who need it appears more distant than ever. Replacing the dream is the specter of a monster—medical care costs are now escalating at two to three times the rate of inflation, the system accords low priority to the predominant health needs of the elderly—the need for chronic illness care in the home and in the community, and it provides instead high cost hospital care that is often inappropriate and unnecessary.

In order to examine the basic issues related to long term care, it is essential that we look at the other side of the coin—acute care as well. It is in solving the problems of acute care that answers can be found for resolving the problems of long term care. The health care cost crisis, as now being socially

Carroll L. Estes is Professor of Sociology and Chairperson of the Department of Social and Behavioral Sciences and Director of the Aging Health Policy Center, School of Nursing, University of California, San Francisco. Dr. Estes conducts research and writes about aging policy, issues in long-term care for the elderly, and the effects of fiscal crisis and new federalism policies on the private, nonprofit sector and on the aging. She is the author of *The Aging Enterprise* (1979) and *The Decision Makers: The Power Structure of Dallas* (1963), and co-author of *Fiscal Austerity and Aging* (1983), *Political Economy, Health, and Aging* (1984), and *Public Policy in Long Term Care* (1984).

315

"constructed" by many of America's most powerful opinion makers, has been defined (erroneously, in my view) as a crisis in excessive consumer demand. Cries of the pending bankruptcy of Medicare are useful political symbols to justify drastic measures—eliminating services, beneficiaries and/or entire programs, while also shifting burdens, costs and responsibilities from government to individuals and their families. The *ideology* underlying the crisis definition is that *the scarcity of resources—rather than human needs—should govern public policy.*

Misunderstandings are created and public support is eroded for health programs when the crisis is defined as the fault of individual elder's choices to use too many health services. This version of the crisis is particularly interesting since it ignores the fact that the doctor admits a patient to the hospital, orders laboratory tests and x-rays, writes the prescriptions and in other ways determines 70–90 percent of medical care costs. There is no evidence that the elderly have misused either Medicare or Medicaid.

Blaming the elderly obscures the fact that rising health costs are directly linked—not to individual abuse of the system—but to the design and financing of Medicare and Medicaid, other public policy choices, as well as the condition of the economy. For example, unemployment reduces payments into Social Security programs; inflation accelerates payments out of the Social Security and Medicare programs; and revenue losses through tax cuts have seriously squeezed health programs.

The abandonment of the goal of access (providing medical care where it is needed), in favor of the goal of cost containment brings us squarely to a critical question: are cost containment and equity inevitable trade-offs?

Some of America's most powerful opinion-makers contend that we are faced with an "either/or" choice between costs and equity in access, that we must accept the consequences like good medicine for the nation's ailing health. A contesting view proposed in this article is that economic efficiency and an equitable, comprehensive health system are not incompatible. The solution lies in a comprehensive approach to health care, not in trying to further fragment an already fragmented system.

The crisis atmosphere that has been generated is fertile

ground for forced and unnecessarily harsh political choices that erode basic entitlements. Nevertheless, the goal of the President's Commission on Ethical Problems in Medicine and Biomedical and Behavioral Research remains an important one—the "ethical obligation to ensure equitable access to health care for all" (U.S. President's Commission, 1983, p. 4).

Given current health policy, those needing long-term care will be faced with a system of restricted access, high costs, often questionable quality, and lack of continuity in care.

BASIC PRINCIPLES OF A COMPREHENSIVE LONG-TERM CARE SYSTEM

An adequate system of long-term care should include seven basic principles:

1. First, it must be comprehensive including a full range of health and social services covering the continuum from community-based care to institutional care.
2. Second, it must be linked with other health and social services as well as acute care services, including hospital care and physician services. (Thus, it must not be separated into its own long-term care closed system.)
3. Third, it must provide incentives for providers to keep costs at a reasonable level, to prevent overutilization and to promote the use of appropriate services.
4. Fourth, it must have a *financing* system that provides protection from the impoverishment of individuals and that allows for combining private and public resources (e.g., allows individuals to buy protection before they become ill and provides coverage for the uninsured).
5. Fifth, it must ensure open access to those who need the services, regardless of ability to pay or other characteristics.
6. Sixth, clients must have access to the services regardless of age. While long-term care is predominantly used by older individuals, it is a system for those of all ages who are disabled. In my view, no adequate rationale for age segregation can be made—age integrated services are critical.

7. Seventh, it must include preventive and restorative services as well as treatment and illness management.

In order to meet these basic principles of a long-term care system, however, several crucial problems must be resolved:

—controlling the overall rate of increase in health care costs (e.g., through such mechanisms as all-payor regulation at the state level, global budgets for hospitals, negotiated fee schedules for physicians);
—developing pooled coverage for those 26 million (or more) Americans who are unable to afford health insurance; and
—establishing incentives for non-hospital acute care services and for community-based, long-term care services.

Researchers, providers, policymakers, families and the concerned public are aware of the high cost and low satisfaction associated with the delivery and organization of long-term care. Some families find themselves in a near desperate state, in some cases, even forced to abandon their elders; some hard-working middle-class retired couples are forced into poverty when one spouse becomes seriously ill; policymakers are talking about increasing family responsibility. The current system is keyed to "helping" long-term patients by institutionalizing and impoverishing them in segregated warehouses for the poor and dying.

Over the past decade the notion of a "continuum of care" which would integrate social and health service systems in order to address both acute and chronic needs, has been articulated and advanced in different ways. Despite impressive accomplishments in geriatric education, technology, and service demonstrations, the truth is that our system performs far below its capacity—and far below that of our neighbor to the north—Canada.

The need to do something is all the more urgent in light of government cutbacks. The monetary and human costs are enormous and must involve all of us in moving in the direction of a viable long-term care strategy, and not merely by piecemeal measures. Where do we begin?

First, we must start with a basic commitment to the notion that chronic illness cannot be separated into certain specific kinds of providers and paid for on a piece-work (fee-for-service) basis. Those with chronic illness not only need the long-term care services, but also they need hospital services, ambulatory medical services, drugs, eyeglasses, podiatry, dental, and many other services that are not traditionally called long-term care services.

Access to this full range of services within one comprehensive system is essential. But can we get there? How have others gotten there? How have the Canadians managed to have a system of comprehensive universal national health insurance—including long-term care at a cost far below that of our fragmented and inadequate system? While a few need to be reminded about the primary issue of cost control in an age of austerity, it must be underscored that the two systems of care (chronic and acute services) are independent. We must have a system that is both age-integrated and service-integrated. Although an integrative approach to long-term care issues and options goes against the current fragmented sources of funding, we must begin to work together on these two fronts. Until we have effective cost control of institutional (especially hospital and nursing home) services, we will not have the capacity to move toward the kind of rational, comprehensive health care system that is needed including long-term care.

Numerous proposals for controlling health care costs are widely debated with enormous vested political and economic interests at stake. Rather than give a detailed explication of complicated formulas, some important features of three proposed strategies of cost control will be highlighted: (1) reimbursement policies, (2) change in the organization of delivery and payment and (3) cost-sharing.

METHODS FOR CONTROLLING HEALTH CARE COSTS

1. Hospital Reimbursement

Because there is general agreement that the rapid rate of increase of health care costs must be reduced, high priority is being given to hospital cost containment through altered reimbursement policies. Congress altered Medicare hospital reimbursement substantially in the Tax Equity and Fiscal Responsibility Act of 1982 and in the 1983 Social Security Amendments. In addition, the Administration has proposed further dramatic increases in patient cost sharing. While this piecemeal approach may reduce hospital expenditures in the Medicare program in the short run, many expect it will result in cost shifting to private third parties unless policies are adopted to prevent that practice by hospitals. Both access and quality of care for the elderly are likely to be diminished *unless the Medicare cost containment policies are part of a cost containment effort that includes all payors.* Unless the rising costs of health care are contained—across the board for hospitals, physicians, nursing homes and even for home health providers, including for all payors, Medicare, Blue Cross, commercial insurance, Medicaid, and other third parties— there will be a continued hemorrhage of Medicare trust funds and this will result in continued rising costs in services and the shifting of these costs to the aged. Medicare cannot be saved by incremental "Medicare only" reforms, no matter how desirable. An "all-payor" hospital reimbursement system has been adopted in four states—New York, New Jersey, Massachusetts, and Maryland. Each state has taken a different approach to regulating hospital payments (e.g., New York has established a per diem rate, New Jersey a per admission rate). Congress must adopt legislation requiring effective cost containment at the state level, and if this is not accomplished, federal regulatory policies must be put into effect.

An example of a method of an all-payor regulation that reaches beyond Medicare-funded services is global budgeting in which government sets limits on the annual hospital expenditure increases to a predetermined amount. Canada's experience illustrates what an effective method global budgeting can be in controlling hospital costs. Since the early 1970s, with the exception of the United Kingdom, Canada has been more effective than any other Western industrialized country in controlling health care costs. Prior to 1971, when Canada's publicly funded medical and hospital insurance program was fully implemented, expenditures had been rising more rapidly in Canada than in the United States (Marmor, 1982; Simanis & Coleman, 1980). Since 1981, however, Canadian health expenditures have been contained to a remarkable degree (in

1971, 7.5 percent of the Canadian GNP was attributed to health expenditures; in 1981, this figure was 7.9 percent; and in 1982, it was approximately 8.2 percent of the GNP). In the United States during the same period, health expenditures rose as a percent of the GNP from 7.8 percent in 1971 to 9.8 percent in 1981 and by 1982, to 10.5 percent. Canada has controlled costs by instituting global hospital budgeting and negotiated fee schedules for physicians (on a fee-for-service basis) at the provincial level.

2. Change in the Organization of Delivery and Payment

In addition to the federal-state role in setting limits on the amount reimbursed for health care, there is also the consideration of potential federal-state government incentives for the way in which health care is organized and reimbursed.

The optimal long-term care system should be built on an incentive structure that encourages providers to control their costs. Prepaid plans are one means of doing this. Preferred provider contracts offer another. One alternative that should be considered is a prepaid and capitated system that permits payment levels to be established in advance of service provision and that bases payment on each individual enrolled rather than on the units of service delivered. This capitated prepayment method, to ensure that providers have incentives to keep costs below the rate provided, has been a key feature of health maintenance organizations which generally have been able to reduce costs to the states where they have been utilized.

Several long-term care programs have developed on this model, that stress social services in addition to Medical services. Called social health maintenance organizations (S/HMOs), a comprehensive delivery system is combined with a financing system that controls costs (Diamond & Berman, 1981). With the addition of long-term care and social service benefits (not included in most HMO plans), S/HMOs are financed with a payment system based on capitation rates (fixed in advance per individual) similar to HMOs. Clients enroll voluntarily, and payments for enrollment may come from a variety of sources including Medicare, Medicaid, and private sources. Initial S/HMOs have been primarily focused on the aged but can serve blind and disabled population groups as well. Strong arguments can be made for offering enrollment to all individuals at risk of disability. S/HMOs are financially "at risk" in that they must provide all benefits for the fixed, prepaid fee. Since costs that are expended over revenues must be covered by the S/HMO, the system is designed to encourage cost-effective management of care.

3. Cost-Sharing

Let us turn now to the differential sacrifice demanded of the major pro-competition health strategy—namely, increased cost-sharing. Escalating health care costs and budget cuts significantly raised the proportion of costs personally shouldered by Medicare recipients in the past four years. Recent policy changes have increased the fiscal hardship for millions of near-poor and poor elderly who are being called upon to bear the growing burden of their health care costs—costs that comprise 17–29 percent of the elderly's budget (except for older white men) and that now exceed $1,430 per capita in out-of-pocket expenses in 1983 (Davis, 1982, p. 25). Out-of-pocket health care expenses are disproportionately borne by older blacks and women (Table 1). These costs are sobering in view of the fact that the median income for individual elders in 1980 was $4,226 (Storey, 1983), and in view of the fact that the poor and minorities tend to be sicker.

Medicare deductibles (the base amount one pays before care becomes covered) and copayments (the proportion of total charges payable by beneficiaries) have both increased dramatically in the past two years. The Part A (Hospital) deductible increased 27 percent between 1981 and 1982 (from $204 to $260), more than double the historical increase. Yet two other increases have been incurred (in 1983, to $304 and 1984, to $356). The medical insurance benefits (Part B physician services) annual deductible rose from $60 in 1981 to $75 in 1982. In addition, the Part B premium, which was $14.60 a month in 1983 is expected to rise to $21.30 a month by 1987, since Congress passed at temporary requirement for Part B premiums to cover 25% of the program costs (Medicare Medicaid Information, 1984, p. 3).

When applied equally to all Medicare beneficiaries, the dif-

Table 1

IMPACT OF DIFFERENT OUT-OF-POCKET HEALTH CARE EXPENDITURES
ON THE MEAN INCOME OF VARIOUS ELDERLY SUBGROUPS, 1981

1981 Per Capita Out-of-Pocket Health Expenditures of the Elderly: $1,154

  o Percent of Mean Income for all Older Persons (13%)
  o Percent of Mean Income for Older Women (17%)
  o Percent of Mean Income for Older Blacks (23%)
  o Percent of Mean Income for Older Black Women (27%)

1981 Per Capita Out-of-Pocket Health Expenditures, Less Nursing
Home Costs, for the Non-Institutionalized Elderly Population: $ 834

  o Percent of Mean Income for All Older Persons (9.5%)
  o Percent of Mean Income for Older Women (12.5%)
  o Percent of Mean Income for Older Blacks (16.5%)
  o Percent of Mean Income for Older Black Women (19.8%)

SOURCE: New York State Office on Aging, 1983.

ferential impact of these flat-rate cost increases becomes clear. As a percentage of income, lower-income elders bear a significantly higher proportionate cost for their health care than do higher-income elders. For example, the Congressional Budget Office projects that "by 1984 noninstitutionalized persons with household incomes under $5,000 will have medical expenditures totalling 97 percent of their $3,659 average income, 18 percent of which they must pay out-of-pocket. Those in the highest income category—of $58,306—will pay just over one percent of their income out-of-pocket" (U.S. CBO, 1983, p. 21).

The increases in copayments and deductibles are expected not only to increase the out-of-pocket payments for the aged, but also to: (1) increase the number of aged who cannot afford to purchase Part B Medicare coverage for physician services; and (2) increase the price of supplemental insurance so that many aged will not be able to purchase it. Both of these changes will further increase costs and inaccessibility to the aged. The small increase in coverage that the Administration has proposed for catastrophic insurance would not offset any of these increased costs to the elderly for Medicare, since estimates are that only two percent of older persons would benefit from the catastrophic coverage (Harrington, 1983).

In summary, the link between the crisis in medical care costs and long-term care for the elderly indicates the need for comprehensive reform of the entire health care system rather than stop-gap measures that penalize those who need medical care the most—the poor and sick.

CONCLUSION

Thus far public policies have addressed short-range approaches to long-term care issues but if Congress or other public policy makers are to entertain the idea of fundamental reform, a long-range perspective is needed.

The goal of an equitable allocation and distribution of the nation's health care resources cannot be reached without a vital federal role in health and aging. As state and local governments across the country devise ways to meet the countervailing demands of taxpayers, providers, and health advocates, it becomes increasingly clear that long-range comprehensive reform will not develop without concerted national leadership.

The Reagan administration's new federalism and decentralization strategy is intended to turn the nation's compass in quite the opposite direction. In framing a long-term care strategy Congress must consider the relationship between state-local government capacity to assume responsibility for the elderly (and particularly for the long-term care policies for the near-poor and poor elderly) and the fiscal context within which state and local governments are operating, the interrelationship between state and federal economic conditions and policies, and the real (and growing) revenue disparities among different states and geographic regions.

The myriad of state-level cost savings strategies in health have not lead to systemwide reform. The research of the Aging Health Policy Center at the University of California, San Francisco, demonstrates that, on the contrary, savings from direct cutbacks or from eligibility restrictions have not resulted in the transfer of money to social and community-based services (Estes, Newcomer & Associates, 1983). Often such savings (when they occur) merely enable state and local governments to keep pace with the overall inflation in medical care prices and the pressures on Medicaid generated by unemployment.

Our society's basic complacency about the notion of a dual policy in health care needs to be challenged. The United States has separate systems of financing and administration for those requiring acute care and for those requiring chronic care. The needs of the patient for acute or chronic illness care cannot easily be separated and the effects of illness can be financially devastating. The idea that hard-working middle and upper-class people will be spared the same indignity of welfare medicine in old age that the poor receive is a myth. Even for those individuals and families living on moderate and middle incomes, expenses for chronic or acute illness can lead to impoverishment. Because private insurance and Medicare do not provide for long-term care coverage, all of us, as we reach old age are at risk of impoverishment in old age without an adequate system of long-term care financing. Who among us could afford the $50 to $100 a day for nursing home care or intensive home care, or $18,000 to $30,000 per year in costs for nursing home care for any extended period of time without losing our home, impoverishing our spouse, and virtually forfeiting an independent and dignified future?

The demand for a solution to the human and economic dilemma of long-term care policy will not be abated by the political call for unequal sacrifice, nor by piecemeal cost control schemes. Nor will the long-term care dilemma be resolved by the Reagan administration's decentralization strategy. Indeed, *an important issue for long-term care policy is the recognition that increasing decentralization of programs for the poor, aged and disabled fosters politically motivated, rather than need-based, priorities and allocations.* The decentralized programs of Medicaid and SSI supplementation have created wide variations in income and health eligibility and benefits for the poor, elderly, blind, and disabled across the states. Due to the stringency of eligibility across the states, less than 50 percent of those below poverty are eligible for Medicaid. Given the current structure of programs relevant to long-term care, US "national" policy is now comprised of multiple, variable, non-comparable policies and programs that are different in different states.

Currently, options for alternative long-term care benefits are heavily influenced by a state's willingness to underwrite the costs. We may recall that Reagan's initial new federalism "swap proposal," which designated complete financial responsibility for long-term care to the hands of state governments, was unanimously and vigorously rejected by the National Governor's Association. Studies of Medicaid, focused on the 1982–83 period, show that most of the state Medicaid policy changes in 1982 were cost-containment strategies aimed at reducing the growth rate in program spending (Estes, Newcomer & Associates, 1983).

These studies further illustrate the vulnerability of the aged to capricious and complex federal and state health and aging policies, as well as to broader policy considerations, such as cost containment and new federalism. These policies have serious consequences for the elderly in this period of inflation and fiscal stress. An exacerbation of the already existing inequities among states is expected in the eligibility and scope of services available to the most disadvantaged elderly.

A major question is whether or not particular long-term policy goals and priorities should be determined nationally or left to the vagaries of state or local politics. Given the structure of current programs, a complete understanding of "national" policy on health care for the aged cannot be obtained without a systematic examination of policies across states. The goal of such an examination should be to distinguish those responsibilities that are logically state and local in nature from those that are so significant in impact that the inequities likely to arise from such decentralized decision making must be prevented through the development of a single national policy.

Numerous proposals have been advanced concerning the need for a uniform national policy on long-term care. Bruce Vladeck's proposal, for example, was to merge Medicare and Medicaid's long-term care portions together into one single continuum of care system (Vladeck, 1981). The private out-of-pocket money spent on long-term care in addition to the Medicaid national long-term care dollar is an enormous sum. A combination of these separate public and private resources might build towards the development of a truly national health insurance protection for older people in this country.

National policy is needed to give all the people of the United States the same kind of universal comprehensive health insurance, including long-term care, that is already enjoyed by our less affluent but equally hard working neighbors to the north—the Canadians. Congress took a major step in enacting Medicare and Medicaid in 1965. We need to go the rest of the way.

REFERENCES

Davis, K. (1982, March). Medicare reconsidered. Paper presented for the Duke University Medical Center Seventh Private Sector Conference on the Financial Support of Health Care of the Elderly and the Indigent, Durham, NC.

Diamond, L. M., & Berman, D. E. (1981). The social/health maintenance organization: A single entry, prepaid, long-term care delivery system. In James J. Callahan & Stanley S. Wallace (Eds.), *Reforming the Long Term Care System*. Lexington, MA: Lexington/Heath.

Estes, C. L. Newcomer, R. J., & Associates. (1983). *Fiscal austerity and aging*. Beverly Hills, CA: Sage, 1983.

Harrington, C. (1983). Social Security and Medicare: Policy shifts in the 1980s. In Estes, Newcomer & Associates, *Fiscal Austerity and Aging: Shifting Government Responsibility for the Elderly*. Beverly Hills, CA: Sage.

Medicare Medicaid Information. (1984, June 26). Congress Finally Agrees to Medicare Cuts. *Medicare Medicaid Information, 9* (10–11), 2–5.

Marmor, T. R. (1982). Is health care better in Canada than in the United States? The view from America. Unpublished paper. New Haven, CT: Yale University.

Simanis, J. D., & Coleman, J. R. (1980, January). Health care expenditures in nine industrialized countries, 1960–1976. *Social Security Bulletin, 43* (1), 3–8.

Storey, J. R. (1983). *Older Americans in the Reagan era: Impacts of federal policy changes.* Washington, DC: Urban Institute.

U.S. Congressional Budget Office (CBO). (1983). *Changing the Structure of Medicare Benefits: Issues and Options.* Washington, DC: U.S. CBO.

U.S. President's Commission for the Study of Ethical Problems in Medicine and Biomedical and Behavioral Research. (1983). *Securing access to health care: A report on the ethical implications of differences in the availability of health services.* Vol. 1: Report. Washington, DC: U.S. Government Printing Office.

Vladeck, B. C. (1981, December). Equity, access, and the costs of health services. *Medical Care, 19*(12), suppl., 69–80.

Vladeck, B. C. (1983). Long term care. Unpublished speech presented to Western Gerontological Society, San Francisco, CA.

CONCLUSION

Long-Term Care: Some Lessons from Cross-National Comparisons

Laura Reif, RN, PhD

When surveying the international scene, one is struck with the similarities across nations in the problems and challenges they face when attempting to organize and finance long-term care. Industrialized nations confront a similar set of conditions: steady growth in the numbers and percentage of the population who have enduring impairments associated with chronic physical and mental diseases; rapidly escalating expenditures related to the care of these persons; and limited resources with which to pay for and deliver the long-term services required. These countries share one further problem: their existing service systems are not optimally designed to deal with the complex, and rapidly-fluctuating needs of the chronically ill and disabled. Furthermore, only limited knowledge is available, so policy-makers and service-planners must often operate without adequate information about either the dimensions of the problem or the effects and costs of alternative solutions.

Laura Reif is Associate Professor in the Department of Family Health Care Nursing at the University of California, San Francisco. She is co-editor of *Home Health Care Services Quarterly*.

COMMON PROBLEMS FACED
BY INDUSTRIALIZED NATIONS

Funding Limitations

A key problem for developed nations is how to provide and pay for the services that are needed by the growing numbers of chronically ill and impaired in all age groups. In most countries, the rapid increase in expenditures for long-term health and social services is a source of great concern. It is difficult to accommodate this increase when public funding is limited. Yet, in most nations, there is growing recognition that both the availability of funding, and the manner in which that money is used, are of critical importance. The amount of funding allocated, the type of service pattern that those funds support, and who is entitled to publicly-financed care—all these factors have a profound effect on the development of services, the continued availability of the organizations and personnel that provide care, and the accessibility of different forms of assistance for populations in need. In short, funding ultimately determines who shall receive services, the amount and type of help given, and the length of time assistance will be continued. A major challenge for industralized nations is how to provide needed long-term care, without outstripping financial resources.

Inadequacy of Existing Service Systems

Within the past decade, many industrialized nations have made substantial progress in redesigning their existing service-network to better accommodate the needs of an increasingly elderly and disabled population. Despite this, several critical problems remain unresolved. Among the most prevalent and intractable of these difficulties are the following:

(1) *Non-uniform access, and lack of universal entitlement to services.* A major problem in many nations is that access to long-term care is not guaranteed to all populations who require this type of assistance. The most notable example of limited access occurs in the United States, where eligibility for publicly-financed long-term care varies, depending on a person's age, income, geographic location, type of illness or disa-

bility, and whether he or she qualifies for care in a specific kind of service-setting. However, even countries with a more enlightened policy of public assistance suffer from similar problems. For example, in France and Sweden, access to social-support services (critical to maintaining chronically ill and disabled at home) differs considerably from region to region, since service provision is largely determined by local authorities, and varies with the resources available in that geographic district. The issue of uniform access to long-term care is a significant one, since unless access is assured (often through the development of adequate mechanisms for financing care), nations will not be fully successful in protecting the chronically ill and aged from impoverishment, unwarranted disability, and premature death.

(2) *Fragmentation of services.* The different elements essential to the provision of long-term care are still fragmented in most nations. Persons who are chronically ill and disabled require a large range of health and social services, housing (often specially-modified to compensate for impairments), income-subsidies, and help with transportation. In industrialized nations, these essential components must still be assembled and coordinated by either professionals or families, who need to draw on the resources of many different service organizations, funding sources, and governmental authorities to assure a comprehensive approach to care.

Divisions between health and social services, between acute and chronic medical care, and between different types of care-settings are very prevalent, even in countries that possess a well-developed range of resources for populations in need of long-term care. None of the industrialized nations has been successful in developing a well-integrated system for delivering long-term assistance to the chronically ill and disabled. In every country there exist gaps—and absence of these essential components within the spectrum of care results in a spill-over of needy individuals into other service sectors. This, in turn, leads to inappropriate use, and often, to excessive costs.

For example, in the United States, underdevelopment and underfunding of in-home social-supportive services (help with housekeeping, meal-preparation, and personal care) has resulted in excessive use of acute-care hospitals and premature placement of many individuals in nursing homes. In Sweden, failure to provide adequate medical services in conjunction with other forms of help in the home, is partly responsible for the "bed-blocking" that occurs when individuals who need long-term assistance must come to the hospital for care.

(3) *Absence of effective mechanisms for matching patients and services, adjusting care over time, and coordinating various types of assistance.* Because services in most countries are fragmented, there is no guarantee that the type of assistance an individual receives will be appropriate. The form of help that is provided is often determined by the extent to which different options are known about and considered, the availability of various types of services, the degree to which a particular service can be paid for (either through public finances or private resources), and, to some extent, the preferences and desires of care-recipients, families, and service-providers.

Specific mechanisms are required to assure that there is a comprehensive assessment of need; that services will be appropriately matched to need; that the type of assistance provided will be revised when there is a change in the health, functional status, living circumstances, or resources of the person who is receiving long-term care; and that services will be coordinated to prevent duplication of effort, conflicting approaches to care, and over- or under-utilization of services. Such mechanisms are still not very well developed in most countries, although some nations have used existing structures to accomplish some of these functions. For example, in the United Kingdom, general practitioners and district health nurses, organized as primary care teams, often serve as service-brokers and care-coordinators for residents in a particular geographical area.

(4) *Inadequate numbers of trained personnel.* Most countries face yet another problem that hampers the effective delivery of long-term services: shortages of trained personnel are very commonplace. This problem is particularly pronounced in countries like the United States, where work with elderly and disabled populations is devalued, chronic care (particularly nursing home care) is poorly funded, and where salary scales, status, and chances for advancement are much lower for personnel providing long-term care than for those involved in the delivery of medical services to persons suffering from acute illnesses. However, shortage of trained person-

nel is a problem which all nations are likely to face in the future, since the rapid growth in the population that needs long-term care can easily lead to a situation in which demand outstrips a country's ability to recruit and train the necessary personnel.

In many countries, ensuring a supply of properly-prepared workers is no mean feat, since existing training programs often fail to provide the knowledge and skills required by those who will care for populations in need of long-term care. For example, conventional doctor- or nurse-training programs emphasize diagnosis of disease, medical intervention, short-term services for the acutely ill, and specialization in a particular category of diseases. In the future, the most pressing need will be for professionals who are generalists, interdisciplinary team members, and care-coordinators. Professionals will need to be able to deal with persons with multiple illnesses, and significant, long-lasting impairments that are not amenable to exclusively-medical interventions. The focus will be on preserving and restoring functional abilities, and on arranging a wide range of supportive services for persons who cannot manage independently because of severe mental or physical deficits. A substantial restructuring of educational programs is necessary to ensure that future generations of professionals will be prepared to approach care from this broader perspective.

Heavy Reliance on the Family as Provider of Long-Term Care

In most countries, an informal support structure of family and friends provides the bulk of daily assistance to chronically ill and impaired persons of all ages. Numerous studies, including one in this volume, have documented the very heavy burden shouldered by family care-givers. There is a growing recognition not only of the importance of help provided by family members, but also of the family's need for support, and for respite from care-taking responsibilities. Countries such as the United Kingdom and France have long-standing traditions of supplying assistance to families who are caring for a sick or disabled member. These countries provide both help in the home and family-respite care (arranging temporary care for the sick person in a hospital, so families can have some relief from the burden of constant care-taking). Some countries provide subsidies to family care-givers. For example, in Sweden, if a family provides assistance to a relative who would ordinarily require services from a home help (nurse's aide), that family is entitled to receive an amount equal to the cost of supplying that personnel.

Despite the existence of these assistance programs, families with impaired or disabled members remain overburdened. The problem will become more pronounced in the future, because of the rapid growth in the numbers of impaired aged and disabled, and the marked decrease in family members available to undertake care-taking responsibilities (family size is decreasing, more women are returning to work, and four-generation families—with multiple elderly and frail members—are more and more common).

Limited Knowledge to Guide Policy and Planning for Long-Term Care

Most countries are hampered by a lack of adequate information on the dimensions of the problems created by the need for long-term services, and the effects and costs of alternative approaches to solving these problems. Indeed, few countries have accurate and complete data on the characteristics of those persons who presently receive long-term assistance; the amount, type and duration of services used; and the total costs of all forms of help provided to this population. Three major problems make it difficult to obtain an adequate data-base: (1) most nations have no systematic and universal scheme for data-reporting that would make it possible to obtain information about care-recipients and service use in different service sectors, and across government programs and jurisdictions (local, regional, national); (2) implementing such a scheme is very problematic because it is difficult to track the movement of care-recipients among assistance programs, and from one service setting to another; and (3) even if an accurate picture of current care-recipients, service use, and costs *could* be obtained, planners would still lack adequate information about the extent of unmet need, and what service utilization and expenditures would look like if services were matched to need, rather than being constrained by inadequate funding and limited availability of services.

There is even less information about the effects and costs of *alternative* approaches to providing help to persons who suffer from serious and long-lasting impairments. In most countries, there is growing recognition that existing resources are not being optimally deployed when managing populations who require long-term care. Yet, information is still relatively limited on the consequences of using different types of service packages, the relative benefits and costs of care provided in different settings (for example, at home versus in a nursing home), and the advantages and disadvantages of new, as opposed to current, models for organizing and delivering services.

Slow Progress in Developing Effective Mechanisms for Containing Costs and for Ensuring the Best Value for Expenditures

The currently-high and ever-increasing expenditures for long-term care are a source of great concern for most nations. Given limited resources for publicly-financed care, a major problem is how to get the most out of money spent on long-term care. While in most countries, the emphasis has been on making available resources go farther, some nations have focused almost exclusively on holding down costs or trying to reduce the amount of money spent on the impaired elderly, the disabled, and other populations needing long-term care. In most nations, only limited progress has been made in developing and successfully implementing strategies for assuring that public funding is used to best effect.

Narrowly-conceived cost-containment efforts have, at times, had some ironic consequences. For example, in the United States, attempts to reduce or cap spending for a particular type of long-term care have often resulted in inappropriate use of more-costly services, and thus *higher* over-all expenditures. Efforts to limit public spending may have tragic consequences as well. It is an easy matter to place strict limits on the amount spent by government for a particular program or service, but funding reductions may lead to such serious problems as increased disability and even premature death among persons who are denied access to essential care.

Lack of a Cohesive National Policy for Long-Term Care

Many countries have yet to articulate a nation-wide policy that spells out how assistance will be provided for persons who have long-term impairments as a result of serious illnesses or injuries. Some countries (such as France, the United Kingdom and Sweden) which have long-standing traditions for publicly-funded health and social services, are adjusting policies and programs to better accommodate the needs of their growing population of impaired elderly. Other countries, like the United States and Australia, lack a cohesive nation-wide policy for providing long-term care.

National leadership in the development of policy is critical to assure equitable access, adequate and universal standards for care, appropriate use of resources, and a comprehensive, coordinated approach to service-delivery. Yet in most nations, policy pertaining to long-term care still lacks coherence. Separate—and often conflicting—policies are produced by multiple, specialized government programs; different administrative authorities; and a variety of overlapping political jurisdictions. The result is great confusion of responsibility, and often-incoherent policies.

EFFORTS TO IMPROVE THE ORGANIZATION AND FINANCING OF LONG-TERM CARE

In most countries, there is a great deal of effort being spent addressing two important questions: (1) what is the best way to provide care for the growing numbers of the disabled and chronically ill in the population? and (2) what is the most effective approach to dealing with the problem of increasing expenditures for long-term care? The "answers" to these questions vary greatly from nation to nation, depending on government (and ultimately the public's) commitment to providing help to the disabled and aged, the tradition for public-financing of health and social programs, and the extent to which various forms of assistance are available and accessible to the population that requires long-term care. In some countries, there has been a major push to solve the problem of high expenditures for long-term care. This seems to be the case in the United States, where cost-containment is the driving force behind most recent changes in health-care policy.

Approaches to Improving Services

A review of the international literature on innovations in the delivery of long-term services reveals a great variety of approaches to improving care. Among the more interesting efforts are those discussed below.

Increasing Access to Services

Several countries are making an effort to increase access to long-term care by lowering the financial barriers that prevent use of services. Some nations (such as the United Kingdom and France) have approached the problem by expanding entitlements and increasing the range of publicly-financed services. Other countries (such as the United States and Germany) are attempting to encourage the development of private insurance coverage for long-term care.

In addition, some nations are trying to assure greater access to services by encouraging case-finding and early identification of individuals who might benefit from care. The efforts made in the United Kingdom to make sure that impaired elderly and disabled are aware of the benefits to which they are entitled is an example of such an approach.

Improving the Availability of Services

Most countries are trying to assure more appropriate long-term care by expanding the range of services that are available. Almost all industralized nations are trying to redress the imbalance between institutional and non-institutional services by expanding home care and other types of assistance which can be provided to individuals outside of hospitals, nursing homes, and other residential care-settings. Some countries, notably the United Kingdom, are experimenting with alternative care packages—different service combinations thought to provide equivalent care, but through use of different mixes of services and different combinations of care-settings.

Virtually all countries are trying to identify and fill gaps in the spectrum of services, so that persons can receive appropriate care in an appropriate setting. At present, many disabled and impaired elderly are provided with a particular service because it is the only form of help available. In an effort to encourage a more appropriate match between services and need, France and Sweden have recently begun to add more medically-oriented care to the range of support-services delivered in the home; the United States has added adult day health care to the service spectrum.

Improving Coordination of Care

Most countries are actively trying to improve the coordination of care across service sectors and care-settings. Some common approaches include: (a) introduction of case-managers or service-brokers, whose main function is to link patients with needed services, and put together an integrated program of care; (b) use of liaison-staff to ensure a smooth transition for persons moving between service setting (hospital to home, hospital to nursing home, home to hospital or nursing home); (c) the development of consolidated service systems, so a broad range of services can be supplied by a single umbrella organization; and (d) creating innovative arrangements that allow coordination of funding and planning across previously separate, specialized programs (for example in some instances, health and social service monies have been pooled in order to support a more complete and integrated program of help for the impaired elderly).

Providing More Support to Family Care-givers

In most countries, there is an awareness that it is important to supplement and support care provided by the informal network of family members and friends. While in some nations (most notably the United States) there is concern that if formal services are increased, these services will supplant unpaid help supplied by family members, most countries are expanding their efforts to provide assistance to families who care for their chronically ill or impaired relatives. Many nations provide training for care-givers, subsidies to relieve the family of the extra financial burden, help in the home which supplements care provided by family members, and respite care in day hospitals and long-stay institutions to provide relief for families who otherwise would have to remain in constant attendance.

Approaches to the Problem of High Expenditures

Most developed countries are also giving attention to the problem of the high cost of long-term care. While there are a great variety of approaches to this problem, it is clear that there are two dominant views on the priority that should be assigned to reducing or controlling expenditures on long-term care. In some nations, cost-considerations are dealt with in the broader context of efforts to make long-term care more available and effective. In other countries, cost-containment is viewed as a important goal in its own right.

Ironically, in at least one country that has given priority to cost-containment, strategies that were primarily designed to reduce spending, have actually led to *increased* expenditures, while service-system reforms have proven much more successful in lowering the costs of long-term care. Perhaps this result is not as surprising as it first appears, since efforts to coordinate care across programs and settings have been shown to result in more effective use of resources, less over-utilization of expensive institutional services, and thus a reduction in total costs. In the United States, a recently-completed evaluation of 13 federally-funded demonstrations (designed to test the effectiveness of coordinated community-based long-term services) indicates that a *combination* of service reforms and cost-containment strategies is needed to ensure the best value for expenditures. These innovative projects clearly demonstrate that services are more effective and the cost of care is lower when (1) services are coordinated through a case-manager or provided through a single organization, (2) access to institutional services is carefully controlled (through pre-admission screening), and (3) formal care supplements and supports, rather than supplants, help provided by family and friends.

Given that service-system reform may be the key to controlling costs, it makes sense that many countries have chosen to focus their efforts in this direction. Some nations, such as the United States, have also put in place mechanisms specifically designed to reduce spending on long-term care. Some of these approaches, while they may prove effective in lowering public expenditures, have already been shown to adversely affect persons who are chronically ill and the families who care for them. For example, attempts to curb government spending in the United States have led to such measures as restricting eligibility and service-benefits, rationing care (allowing only certain groups access to services), setting limits on the amount that government will pay for a given service, shifting some of the costs of care to consumers, and requiring families to assume greater responsibility for providing or paying for care of chronically ill or impaired relatives. These cost-containment strategies have resulted in a system of 2-track medical care (with greatly-restricted services and lower-quality care for the poor), a much higher level of out-of-pocket expenditures for the elderly (who now spend more on their medical care than they did prior to the implementation of a government-financed health insurance program for the aged), and increased rates of morbidity, disability and mortality for those who are denied access to services. No rational and humane approach to the problems associated with the high cost of long-term care could be based exclusively on the cost-containment strategies outlined above.

However, one approach to cost-containment (now being tried in the United States) *does* seem to have considerable promise. The core feature of this approach is to require that care-providers take some responsibility for monitoring and, where possible, controlling the costs of the services they deliver. This can be achieved in a variety of ways: (1) assigning a case-manager responsibility for coordinating care and for determining access to services, and requiring that he or she specifically consider costs when recommending a particular package of services for the sick person; (2) paying service-organizations and professionals a pre-determined, negotiated amount for care, rather than continuing to reimburse on the basis of fees that are determined exclusively by providers; and (3) financing services through a pre-paid, capitated system, under which a health-care organization is paid a set fee, in advance, and thereafter is responsible for providing a comprehensive range of medical services to persons who are enrolled in the program.

SUMMARY

A review of how long-term care is provided in a number of industrialized nations, sheds more light on the problem than on the solutions. However, it is clear that the problem of providing adequate assistance to the chronically ill and disabled is universal, that this problem is very difficult to solve, and that it is likely to become worse in the future. A consideration of experiences in different countries amply illustrates that simplistic solutions (such as focusing efforts exclusively on cost-containment) do not work, and may often exacerbate the problem. It is also apparent that, in all countries, a more systematic and comprehensive approach to the problem is not only desirable, but necessary.